AWAKEN THE MIND: A JOURNEY TO MINDFULNESS AND INNER PEACE

Mir M Hossain

ISBN-13: 9798867317232

Cover design by: Art Painter
Library of Congress Control Number: 2018675309
Printed in the United States of America

INTRODUCTION: THE PATH TO INNER PEACE

In a world filled with constant noise, distractions, and the ever-accelerating pace of life, the quest for inner peace has never been more vital. Many of us find ourselves yearning for a sanctuary of serenity amid the chaos. We seek a refuge where the mind can find respite, where the soul can breathe freely, and where the heart can rediscover its rhythm. inner peace is not only a personal state of being but also a means to foster peace and harmony in society. We are encouraged to be peacemakers and work toward resolving conflicts and injustices. The quest for inner peace is intricately connected to the broader goal of creating a just and peaceful world

This book, "Awaken the Mind: A Journey to Mindfulness and Inner Peace," is an invitation to embark on a transformative voyage—one that leads to the heart of mindfulness. Mindfulness is not merely a practice; it is a way of life, a philosophy, and a path to profound inner peace. It is a journey of self-discovery, self-acceptance, and self-compassion. It's a pilgrimage that allows us to uncover the treasures within, connect with the world around us, and unearth the wisdom that resides in the present moment.

Throughout these pages, you'll explore the essence of mindfulness, uncover the intricate connection between your mind and body, and learn how to dwell fully in the present. This book will guide you on the path to understanding the art of mindfulness and the tremendous impact it can have on your life. You'll discover that the journey to inner peace is not just about reaching a destination—it's about savoring the steps along the way. The holistic view of well-being is that the health of the body and the state of the mind are interrelated

As you embrace mindfulness, you'll encounter the power of the present moment, learn to navigate the intricate landscape of your inner world, and foster more meaningful connections with those around you. The path to inner peace is not without its challenges, but the rewards are immeasurable. So, let's embark on this journey together, where every page is a step toward awakening the mind, nurturing inner peace, and embracing the beauty of the present moment. Welcome to a transformative odyssey—an exploration of mindfulness and a quest for inner peace.

CHAPTER 1: MINDFULNESS UNVEILED

What Is Mindfulness ?

Defining Mindfulness in General

Mindfulness is a mental and emotional state characterized by a heightened awareness of the present moment, without judgment or attachment to past or future thoughts and experiences. It involves paying deliberate attention to one's thoughts, feelings, bodily sensations, and the surrounding environment. While rooted in various spiritual and philosophical traditions, mindfulness has gained widespread recognition as a secular practice that offers numerous psychological and health benefits. Key elements of mindfulness include:

Present-Moment Awareness: Mindfulness encourages individuals to focus on what is happening right now, rather than dwelling on the past or worrying about the future. It involves fully immersing oneself in the current experience.

Non-Judgmental Observation: Mindfulness invites a non-judgmental stance toward one's thoughts and emotions. Rather than labeling them as "good" or "bad," individuals observe and accept them as they are.

Acceptance and Tolerance: It involves accepting the reality of the present moment, even if it is challenging or uncomfortable. Mindfulness teaches tolerance and the acknowledgment of the transient nature of emotions and experiences.

Self-Reflection and Self-Awareness: Practicing mindfulness often leads to increased self-awareness. It encourages individuals to explore their own thought patterns, emotional reactions, and behavioral tendencies.

Breath and Body Awareness: Many mindfulness practices incorporate focused attention on the breath and bodily sensations. The body serves as an anchor to the present moment, helping individuals stay grounded.

Emotional Regulation: Mindfulness can aid in emotional regulation, allowing individuals to respond to situations with greater composure and resilience. It fosters emotional intelligence.

Stress Reduction: Mindfulness is widely recognized for its stress-reduction benefits. By staying present and managing reactions to stressors, individuals can experience a greater sense of calm and relaxation.

Improved Concentration: Practicing mindfulness enhances one's ability to concentrate and sustain attention on tasks, leading to increased productivity and performance.

Relationship Enhancement: Mindfulness can improve the quality of interpersonal relationships by promoting active listening, empathy, and a non-reactive, non-judgmental approach to communication.

Spiritual and Transcendental Aspects: In some traditions, mindfulness is considered a spiritual practice that connects individuals to a greater sense of purpose, inner peace, and transcendence.

Mindfulness is often cultivated through various techniques, including meditation, deep breathing exercises, yoga, and other mindfulness practices. It is commonly used in therapeutic contexts, such as Mindfulness-Based Stress Reduction (MBSR) and Mindfulness-Based Cognitive Therapy (MBCT), to help individuals manage a wide range of conditions, from anxiety and depression to chronic pain. Ultimately, mindfulness is a versatile and accessible tool that can lead to a deeper understanding of oneself and a more conscious, intentional way of living.

Historical Roots Of Mindfulness

Mindfulness has deep historical roots, with its origins dating back thousands of years. While it is widely associated with Buddhist and Hindu traditions, the concept of mindfulness transcends religious and cultural boundaries. Here is an overview of its historical development:

Buddhism: Mindfulness, known as "sati" in Pali and "smṛti" in Sanskrit, is a core component of Buddhist teachings. The historical Buddha, Siddhartha Gautama, emphasized mindfulness as a way to attain enlightenment and escape suffering. He encouraged his followers to be fully present in each moment, to observe their thoughts and feelings without attachment, and to cultivate insight into the impermanence of all things. This practice is central to the Four Foundations of Mindfulness (Satipatthana), a key teaching in Buddhism.

Hinduism: Mindfulness is also integral to Hindu philosophy. In the Bhagavad Gita, an important Hindu scripture, the concept of mindfulness is discussed in the context of self-awareness and control over one's mind and senses. It is closely related to the practice of yoga and meditation, which aim to achieve a state of self-realization and union with the divine.

Ancient Greece: Greek philosophers such as Socrates and Aristotle explored the idea of self-awareness and "knowing thyself." They emphasized introspection, self-examination, and self-reflection as means to personal growth and wisdom, concepts that align with mindfulness principles.

Early Christianity: Early Christian mystics and ascetics practiced a form of mindfulness as part of their spiritual journey. The Desert Fathers and Mothers engaged in contemplative practices that involved self-reflection, inner silence, and connection with God.

Islamic View: Mindfulness, known in Arabic as "Taqwa," has deep historical roots within the Islamic tradition. It is a concept and practice that goes beyond mere religious rituals, emphasizing a profound awareness of God (Allah), ethical conduct, and the present moment. The Quran, the holy book of Islam, repeatedly emphasizes mindfulness and the concept of Taqwa. Taqwa is often translated as "mindfulness" or "consciousness of God" and is mentioned throughout the Quran as a means to lead a righteous life. Believers are encouraged to be mindful of God's presence, commands, and ethical principles in their daily actions

Mindfulness in Judaism: Jewish meditation, known as "hitbodedut" or "hisbonenus," has been practiced for centuries. It involves introspection, self-reflection, and the cultivation of a deeper connection with God. Meditation allows individuals to focus on their thoughts, feelings, and the Divine presence in their lives.

Zen Buddhism: In Zen Buddhism, mindfulness takes the form of "zazen," or seated meditation. Zen practitioners focus on the breath and the present moment as a means of attaining insight and enlightenment. Zen mindfulness has had a significant influence on the development of mindfulness practices in the West.

Secular Mindfulness: In the 20th and 21st centuries, mindfulness has gained popularity as a secular practice, divorced from its religious or philosophical roots. Jon Kabat-Zinn is credited with introducing Mindfulness-Based Stress Reduction (MBSR) in the late 1970s, which has since been used in clinical and therapeutic settings. Similarly, Mindfulness-Based Cognitive Therapy (MBCT) combines cognitive therapy with mindfulness practices to treat conditions like depression and anxiety.

Modern Applications: Today, mindfulness is widely embraced for its therapeutic and psychological benefits. It is used in various contexts, including education, healthcare, corporate settings, and stress reduction programs. Mindfulness practices have become part of mainstream wellness and self-care.

The historical roots of mindfulness illustrate its universal and enduring appeal as a means of self-awareness, inner peace, and personal growth. While its origins are diverse, the core principles of being present, non-judgmental, and self-aware remain consistent across time and cultures.

The Modern Relevance Of Mindfulness

In today's fast-paced and often stress-filled world, the practice of mindfulness has gained significant modern relevance. It offers a wide range of benefits for individuals, communities, and society as a whole. Here are some key aspects of the modern relevance of mindfulness:

Stress Reduction: Mindfulness is widely recognized for its ability to reduce stress and promote emotional well-being. In an era marked by high levels of stress and anxiety, mindfulness practices offer practical techniques to manage and alleviate these challenges.

Mental Health: Mindfulness-based interventions, such as Mindfulness-Based Stress Reduction (MBSR) and Mindfulness-Based Cognitive Therapy (MBCT), have shown effectiveness in addressing mental health issues like depression, anxiety, and post-traumatic stress disorder. It has become an integral part of contemporary psychotherapy.

Productivity and Focus: In a world filled with distractions, mindfulness enhances focus and concentration. It helps individuals become more present in their tasks, leading to increased productivity and efficiency.

Emotional Intelligence: Mindfulness promotes emotional intelligence by encouraging individuals to understand, manage, and express their emotions in healthy ways. This is valuable in personal relationships, the workplace, and leadership roles.

Workplace Wellness: Many companies and organizations have adopted mindfulness programs to improve workplace wellness. Mindfulness can reduce employee stress, enhance job satisfaction, and foster a more positive work environment.

Physical Health: The mind-body connection is central to mindfulness. As people become more mindful, they often make healthier lifestyle choices, leading to improved physical health. This can impact areas such as sleep, eating habits, and exercise.

Relationships: Mindfulness practices, including mindful communication and active listening, contribute to healthier and more fulfilling relationships. It helps individuals relate to others with empathy, openness, and less reactivity.

Resilience: Mindfulness helps build resilience by teaching individuals to respond to adversity with equanimity and adaptability. It equips people to bounce back from challenges more effectively.

Reduced Impulsivity: Mindfulness teaches individuals to respond thoughtfully rather than react impulsively. This is valuable in decision-making, conflict resolution, and self-control.

Spiritual Growth: In a secular context, mindfulness is often considered a path to spiritual growth. It offers a way for individuals to explore questions of meaning, purpose, and transcendence.

Global Well-Being: As individuals practice mindfulness and experience its benefits, it contributes to a more peaceful and harmonious society. This extends to a global context, fostering a culture of understanding, empathy, and compassion.

Educational Settings: Mindfulness is increasingly incorporated into educational curricula to enhance student well-being, emotional regulation, and cognitive development. It helps children and young adults cope with academic pressures.

Digital Detox: In an age of constant connectivity, mindfulness serves as a reminder to unplug and find balance. It encourages people to spend time away from screens and reconnect with the physical world.

Crisis Management: Mindfulness practices are used in crisis management and disaster relief to help individuals cope with trauma, grief, and loss. It provides tools for psychological resilience.

Self-Care: Mindfulness is a vital component of self-care. It encourages individuals to prioritize their well-being, engage in self-compassion, and maintain a balanced, healthy life.

The modern relevance of mindfulness lies in its potential to address many of the challenges of contemporary life. It is a versatile and accessible practice that empowers individuals to lead healthier, more balanced, and fulfilling lives in an increasingly complex and fast-paced world.

CHAPTER 2: THE MIND-BODY CONNECTION

Understanding The Mind-Body Link

The mind-body link is a complex and profound connection between mental and physical well-being, where the state of one significantly impacts the other. This connection has been a subject of study and exploration in various fields, including psychology, medicine, and philosophy. Here's an overview of the understanding of the mind-body link:

Psychosomatic Interaction: Psychosomatic interaction refers to the intricate relationship between a person's mental or emotional state and their physical health. The term "psychosomatic" is derived from the Greek words "psyche" (mind) and "soma" (body), highlighting the interplay between psychological and physical aspects of well-being. Understanding psychosomatic interaction is crucial for recognizing how emotional and mental factors can influence physical health. Here are key points to consider:

Mind-Body Connection: Psychosomatic interaction is a prime example of the mind-body connection, where mental and emotional states can have a significant impact on physical health. The mind can influence bodily functions and, conversely, physical conditions can affect one's mental and emotional well-being.

Emotions and Physical Symptoms: Emotional states, such as stress, anxiety, and depression, can manifest as physical symptoms. For example, chronic stress can lead to headaches, muscle tension, digestive issues, and sleep disturbances. These physical symptoms are a direct result of emotional distress.

Somatic Symptom Disorders: Somatic symptom disorders involve excessive worry or preoccupation with physical symptoms. These conditions are rooted in emotional distress and can lead to the development of genuine physical symptoms.

Pain Perception: Psychosomatic factors can influence pain perception. Emotional distress can exacerbate the perception of pain, while a positive emotional state may lead to pain relief or a higher pain tolerance.

Stress and Physical Health: Chronic stress is a prime example of psychosomatic interaction. It triggers the body's stress response, leading to physiological changes like increased heart rate, elevated blood pressure, and the release of stress hormones. Prolonged stress is associated with a range of health problems, from cardiovascular issues to compromised immunity.

Placebo and Nocebo Effects: The placebo effect demonstrates how a person's belief in the effectiveness of a treatment, even if it's inactive, can lead to real health improvements. Conversely, the nocebo effect occurs when a person experiences negative side effects due to negative expectations or beliefs about a treatment.

Resilience and Coping: Psychosomatic factors are essential in understanding resilience and coping mechanisms. Individuals with strong emotional resilience may better manage physical health challenges, while those experiencing emotional distress may find it more difficult to cope with physical ailments.

Psychosomatic Medicine: This medical specialty focuses on the diagnosis and treatment of conditions where psychological factors play a significant role in physical health. Psychosomatic medicine recognizes the importance of addressing both emotional and physical aspects of well-being.

Holistic Health: Holistic approaches to health recognize the mind-body connection and aim to address health issues by considering mental, emotional, and physical factors as interrelated components of overall well-being.

Mind-Body Therapies: Mind-body therapies, such as cognitive-behavioral therapy (CBT) and biofeedback, are designed to help individuals recognize and manage the impact of psychosomatic factors on their health. These therapies provide strategies to address emotional distress that may be contributing to physical symptoms.

Understanding psychosomatic interaction highlights the need for comprehensive health care that considers the whole person. It emphasizes that emotional and mental states can influence physical health and that addressing both aspects is vital for holistic well-being. This recognition is crucial for healthcare professionals, individuals dealing with health challenges, and anyone interested in maintaining a balanced and healthy life.

Stress and Health: Chronic stress can lead to a range of physical health problems, including cardiovascular issues, weakened immune system, and digestive disorders. The body's stress response triggers physiological changes, impacting overall well-being.

Placebo Effect: The placebo effect demonstrates the power of the mind in healing. Belief in the effectiveness of a treatment, even if it is inert, can lead to actual improvements in physical health. This illustrates the mind's influence on the body's healing mechanisms.

Emotions and Immunity: Emotional states, such as happiness and optimism, have been associated with a strengthened immune system. Conversely, negative emotions like chronic stress and depression can weaken immune function.

Mindfulness and Pain Management: Mindfulness practices have proven effective in managing chronic pain. By altering the perception of pain and increasing pain tolerance, individuals can experience relief through mental techniques.

Neurotransmitters and Mood: The brain produces neurotransmitters, such as serotonin and dopamine, which play a crucial role in mood regulation. Imbalances in these neurotransmitters are linked to mental health conditions like depression and anxiety, which can, in turn, affect physical health.

Mind-Body Interventions: Mind-body interventions encompass a range of practices, including yoga, tai chi, and meditation, that foster a deeper connection between the mind and body. These techniques have gained recognition for their profound impact on overall well-being. They bridge the perceived gap between mental and physical health, emphasizing their intrinsic connection. Here's a more detailed exploration of how these practices promote relaxation, reduce stress, and enhance physical health while cultivating a profound sense of balance and well-being:

Yoga: Yoga is a holistic practice that combines physical postures, controlled breathing, and meditation. It encourages individuals to be fully present in the moment, promoting a mindful awareness of the body and breath. Through various poses and stretches, yoga improves flexibility and strength. Simultaneously, it reduces stress and anxiety, promoting emotional well-being. The mind-body connection in yoga is evident as practitioners become more attuned to bodily sensations and emotions, fostering a profound sense of inner balance and peace.

Tai Chi: Tai chi is a martial art characterized by slow, flowing movements and deep breathing. It is often referred to as "moving meditation." Tai chi encourages a deep state of relaxation, which in turn reduces stress. The slow and deliberate movements promote balance, coordination, and physical well-being. This practice exemplifies the concept of "qi" or "chi," which signifies the life force energy that flows through the body. By fostering a harmonious flow of energy, tai chi strengthens the mind-body connection.

Meditation: Meditation comes in various forms, all of which involve a deliberate focus on the present moment. Whether it's mindfulness meditation, loving-kindness meditation, or transcendental meditation, the goal is to quiet the mind, reduce stress, and cultivate inner peace. Through meditation, individuals become more aware of their thoughts, emotions, and physical sensations. This heightened awareness allows them to release stress and tension, leading to enhanced physical and emotional health.

Relaxation Response: Mind-body interventions trigger what Herbert Benson, a pioneer in mind-body medicine, termed the "relaxation response." This is the body's opposite reaction to the stress-induced "fight-or-flight" response. The relaxation response induces a state of deep relaxation, slowing heart rate, lowering blood pressure, and promoting a sense of calm. By consistently eliciting the relaxation response through mind-body practices, individuals can reduce the detrimental effects of chronic stress on their physical and mental health.

Balanced Well-Being: The common thread among these practices is their ability to promote a sense of balance and well-being. They encourage individuals to find equilibrium within themselves, harmonizing the mental and physical aspects of health. By embracing the mind-body connection, these interventions help individuals maintain a state of holistic health where physical vitality and emotional serenity coexist.

Psychoneuroimmunology: This interdisciplinary field studies the relationship between psychological factors, the nervous system, and the immune system. It explores how mental states can impact immune responses and vulnerability to diseases.

The Gut-Brain Connection: The gut-brain axis demonstrates the bidirectional communication between the gastrointestinal system and the brain. Gut health has been linked to mental health, and conditions like irritable bowel syndrome (IBS) can be exacerbated by stress.

Biofeedback and Mental Control: Biofeedback techniques enable individuals to gain conscious control over physiological processes like heart rate, blood pressure, and muscle tension. By learning to control these functions, people can improve mental and physical health.

Mind-Body Therapies: Therapies like cognitive-behavioral therapy (CBT) address the mind-body link by helping individuals recognize and change negative thought patterns that can lead to emotional distress and physical symptoms.

Epigenetics: Epigenetics explores how environmental factors, including psychological stress, can influence gene expression. It reveals that mental states can leave an epigenetic mark on DNA, affecting physical health.

Holistic Health: Holistic approaches to health emphasize the interconnectedness of mind, body, and spirit. They view health as a whole and recognize that one's mental and emotional state is intertwined with physical well-being.

Understanding the mind-body link underscores the importance of holistic well-being and the interconnectedness of mental and physical health. It highlights the profound impact that thoughts, emotions, and stress can have on the body's functioning and overall health. Promoting mental and emotional well-being is an essential aspect of maintaining a healthy and balanced life.

Mindful Practices For Health And Wellness

Mindful practices play a pivotal role in promoting health and wellness by fostering a profound connection between the mind and body. These practices encourage individuals to be fully present in the moment, reduce stress, and enhance overall well-being. Here are some mindful practices that contribute to health and wellness:

Meditation: Meditation is a versatile practice that comes in various forms, including mindfulness meditation, loving-kindness meditation, and transcendental meditation. It involves focused attention and awareness of the present moment. Regular meditation helps reduce stress, improve emotional regulation, and promote mental clarity, contributing to overall well-being.

Yoga: Yoga is a holistic practice that combines physical postures, breathing techniques, and meditation. It enhances flexibility, strength, and balance while promoting relaxation and reducing anxiety. Yoga fosters a strong mind-body connection and is beneficial for physical and emotional health.

Mindful Eating: Mindful eating is the practice of paying full attention to the experience of eating, savoring each bite and being aware of the sensory qualities of the food. This practice promotes healthy eating habits, prevents overeating, and encourages a deeper appreciation of the nourishment provided by food.

Breathing Exercises: Simple breathing exercises, such as

diaphragmatic breathing and box breathing, help individuals regulate their breath and induce a state of calm. Controlled breathing reduces stress and anxiety, enhances focus, and supports relaxation.

Tai Chi: Tai chi, often referred to as "moving meditation," involves slow, flowing movements combined with deep, controlled breathing. This practice enhances balance, coordination, and flexibility while reducing stress and promoting a sense of inner peace.

Nature Walks: Spending time in nature and taking mindful walks in natural settings can significantly improve mental and physical well-being. Nature walks promote relaxation, reduce stress, and enhance a sense of connection with the environment.

Progressive Muscle Relaxation: This practice involves systematically tensing and relaxing muscle groups to release physical tension. It is effective for reducing muscle tightness, promoting relaxation, and alleviating stress.

Journaling: Keeping a mindfulness journal allows individuals to express their thoughts and emotions in a reflective and non-judgmental way. Journaling can provide clarity, reduce stress, and improve emotional well-being.

Gratitude Practices: Focusing on gratitude involves recognizing and appreciating the positive aspects of life. Gratitude practices, such as keeping a gratitude journal or engaging in daily gratitude reflections, enhance mental and emotional health by fostering a positive outlook.

Body Scan Meditation: The body scan is a mindfulness meditation technique that involves mentally scanning the body from head to toe, paying attention to physical sensations and areas of tension. It promotes relaxation, reduces physical discomfort, and enhances self-awareness.

Loving-Kindness Meditation: This practice involves cultivating feelings of love, compassion, and goodwill toward oneself and others. It fosters emotional well-being, self-compassion, and positive social interactions.

Mindful Movement: Engaging in mindful physical activities, such as walking, jogging, or dancing, with a focus on the present moment and bodily sensations, promotes physical fitness and emotional well-being.

Visualization: Guided visualization exercises encourage individuals to imagine positive scenarios and outcomes. Visualization can reduce stress, enhance confidence, and improve emotional resilience.

These mindful practices are integral to health and wellness, as they empower individuals to nurture their mental and physical well-being. They offer a holistic approach to self-care, emphasizing the importance of maintaining a strong mind-body connection and living in the present moment. Whether through meditation, movement, or reflection, these practices contribute to a balanced and healthy life.

Techniques For Cultivating Mind-Body Harmony

Cultivating mind-body harmony is a profound journey towards holistic well-being, where the interplay between mental and physical health is nurtured. By embracing various techniques, individuals can harmonize their mind and body, fostering a sense of balance, peace, and vitality. Here are techniques that promote mind-body harmony:

Mindfulness Meditation: Mindfulness meditation involves being fully present in the moment, observing thoughts and sensations without judgment. This practice encourages mental clarity, emotional regulation, and a deep connection with the body.

Yoga: Yoga combines physical postures, breathing exercises, and meditation to enhance flexibility, strength, and balance. It fosters a strong mind-body connection, promoting relaxation and reducing stress.

Tai Chi: Tai chi's slow, flowing movements and controlled breathing create a sense of mindfulness in motion. It improves balance, coordination, and overall physical well-being, while reducing stress and anxiety.

Breath Awareness: Conscious breath control, such as diaphragmatic breathing and box breathing, helps individuals regulate their breath, reducing stress and promoting relaxation.

Progressive Muscle Relaxation: This technique involves systematically tensing and releasing muscle groups to release physical tension and promote relaxation.

Biofeedback: Biofeedback provides real-time data on physiological functions like heart rate and muscle tension. By learning to control these functions, individuals can enhance mental and physical well-being.

Body Scan Meditation: The body scan involves mentally scanning the body from head to toe, focusing on physical sensations and areas of tension. This practice promotes relaxation and self-awareness.

Visualization: Guided visualization exercises encourage individuals to imagine positive scenarios and outcomes, fostering emotional resilience and reducing stress.

Loving-Kindness Meditation: Cultivating feelings of love,

compassion, and goodwill toward oneself and others enhances emotional well-being and positive social interactions.

Mindful Eating: Mindful eating practices focus on fully experiencing the sensory qualities of food and savoring each bite. This approach promotes healthy eating habits and emotional balance.

Gratitude Practices: Recognizing and appreciating the positive aspects of life through gratitude practices, like keeping a gratitude journal or daily reflections, fosters a positive outlook and emotional well-being.

Nature Connection: Spending time in nature, practicing mindfulness in natural settings, and engaging in nature walks enhances relaxation and fosters a sense of connection with the environment.

Journaling: Keeping a mindfulness journal allows individuals to express thoughts and emotions in a reflective and non-judgmental manner, promoting emotional clarity and well-being.

Mindful Movement: Engaging in physical activities with a focus on the present moment and bodily sensations, such as walking, jogging, or dancing, enhances physical fitness and emotional well-being.

Holistic Health Practices: Approaches that encompass both mental and physical aspects of health, such as holistic medicine and integrative therapies, emphasize mind-body harmony and overall well-being.

Deep Breathing Techniques: Practicing deep breathing exercises, like the 4-7-8 technique, helps calm the mind and reduce stress, promoting a harmonious balance between mental and physical states.

Holistic Therapies: Therapies such as aromatherapy, acupuncture, and acupressure address both mental and physical well-being, helping to align the mind and body.

Sound Healing: Sound healing practices, like singing bowls or sound baths, promote relaxation and emotional balance by harmonizing the mind and body through sound vibrations.

Traditional Eastern Practices: Drawing from ancient traditions, techniques like Ayurveda and traditional Chinese medicine emphasize the interconnectedness of mental and physical well-being.

Creative Expression: Engaging in creative activities, whether through art, music, or writing, fosters emotional expression and self-awareness, contributing to mind-body harmony.

Cultivating mind-body harmony is a dynamic and evolving journey. By incorporating these techniques into daily life, individuals can achieve a deeper sense of balance, inner peace, and vitality, promoting both mental and physical well-being.

CHAPTER 3: EXAMPLE OF SUCCESSFUL PEOPLE USING MINDULNESS OR LONG LIFE:

here are examples of successful individuals who have embraced mindfulness practices and long, healthy lives as part of their lifestyles:

Oprah Winfrey: Media mogul Oprah Winfrey has openly endorsed mindfulness and meditation practices as integral to her success and well-being. She introduced the concept of the "Super Soul Sunday" show, which explores spiritual and mindfulness themes. Oprah attributes much of her success to these practices, as they provide her with clarity and a sense of balance.

Richard Branson: The founder of the Virgin Group, Richard Branson, is known for his adventurous spirit and business acumen. He has credited a combination of mindfulness and a balanced lifestyle for his success. Regularly engaging in activities like kite-surfing and meditation, Branson promotes the idea that a sound mind and body are essential for thriving in the business world.

Arianna Huffington: The co-founder of The Huffington Post, Arianna Huffington, is a strong advocate for well-being and mindfulness. After experiencing the negative effects of sleep deprivation, she dedicated herself to promoting a healthier work-life balance. She established Thrive Global, a company focused on improving well-being and productivity through mindfulness practices.

Ray Dalio: The founder of Bridgewater Associates, one of the world's largest hedge funds, Ray Dalio incorporates meditation and mindfulness into his daily routine. He believes that these practices contribute to his decision-making abilities and success in the finance industry.

Steve Jobs: The late co-founder of Apple, Steve Jobs, practiced mindfulness and meditation as a means of enhancing creativity and reducing stress. He often attributed his innovative thinking to these practices and incorporated them into his daily life.

Warren Buffett: Warren Buffett, one of the most successful investors in history, credits his longevity and success to a balanced and mindful lifestyle. He maintains a relatively simple life, emphasizing the importance of managing stress and making deliberate decisions.

Ellen DeGeneres: The beloved television host and comedian, Ellen DeGeneres, practices mindfulness to stay grounded and maintain a positive outlook. She has openly discussed the benefits of meditation and gratitude in her life.

Deepak Chopra: A well-known advocate for holistic health and mindfulness, Deepak Chopra has built a successful career as an author and speaker. He promotes the integration of mind-body practices, including meditation and yoga, for overall well-being and success.

Jane Goodall: Renowned primatologist and conservationist Jane Goodall has dedicated her life to studying and protecting wildlife. Her mindful approach to observing nature and her deep connection to the environment are integral to her success in the field of conservation.

Rupert Murdoch: Media mogul Rupert Murdoch has expressed his interest in mindfulness and meditation as tools for maintaining a balanced and successful life. He believes that these practices help him manage the stress associated with running a global media empire.

These successful individuals from various fields have integrated mindfulness practices and balanced lifestyles into their routines. Their experiences highlight how a focus on mental and physical well-being can contribute to their achievements and longevity.

CHAPTER 4: THE ART OF BEING PRESENT

Living In The Present Moment

Remember, "no amount of guilt can change your past and no amount of Worries can change the future" That's a profound reminder. Guilt and worry are emotions that often pull us away from the present moment. Understanding that dwelling on the past with guilt or being consumed by worries about the future won't alter what has already happened or what's to come is a valuable lesson. Instead, focusing on the present and taking positive actions in the here and now can lead to a more balanced and fulfilling life. It's a reminder to embrace mindfulness and live in the present moment, as it's the only moment where we have the power to make a real difference.

Mindfulness is the practice of intentionally paying full attention to the present moment without judgment. Living in the present moment is at the heart of mindfulness, and it has a profound impact on mental, emotional, and physical well-being. Here's a deeper exploration of the concept:

Awareness of the Now: Mindfulness encourages individuals to be fully aware of the present moment. It involves acknowledging one's thoughts, feelings, bodily sensations, and the environment without dwelling on the past or worrying about the future.

Reducing Stress: Mindfulness helps reduce stress by redirecting focus away from anxious thoughts about the future or regrets about the past. By concentrating on the here and now, individuals can manage stress and anxiety more effectively.

Emotional Regulation: Being present in the moment allows for a more balanced emotional state. Mindfulness helps individuals respond to their emotions with greater clarity, reducing impulsivity and reactivity.

Enhanced Focus: Living in the present moment enhances concentration and cognitive abilities. By concentrating on a single task without distractions, individuals can accomplish more and achieve a greater sense of fulfillment.

Improved Relationships: Mindfulness fosters better relationships by encouraging individuals to be fully present when interacting with others. Listening attentively and empathizing with those around you can lead to stronger connections.

Gratitude: Living in the present moment promotes gratitude by allowing individuals to recognize and appreciate the beauty and opportunities of the current moment.

Reduced Rumination: Rumination, or repetitive thinking about negative experiences, is diminished through mindfulness. By staying present, individuals can break the cycle of overthinking.

Physical Benefits: Mindfulness can have physical benefits, such as reducing blood pressure, improving sleep quality, and enhancing overall well-being.

Enhanced Creativity: Living in the present moment can stimulate creativity and problem-solving skills. It encourages a fresh perspective on challenges and opportunities.

Self-Discovery: Mindfulness allows for a deeper understanding of oneself, including values, priorities, and goals. It promotes self-discovery and personal growth.

Mind-Body Connection: Mindfulness practices bridge the gap between mental and physical well-being. They encourage individuals to recognize how thoughts and emotions can influence physical sensations and health.

Mindful Activities: Everyday activities can be approached mindfully, such as eating, walking, and even breathing. Engaging in these activities with full awareness can enhance the quality of experiences.

Acceptance and Non-Judgment: Mindfulness emphasizes acceptance of the present moment without judgment. It allows individuals to observe their experiences without labeling them as good or bad.

Living in the present moment is a fundamental aspect of mindfulness. It enables individuals to experience life more fully, reduce stress, enhance emotional well-being, and improve physical health. By embracing mindfulness practices and the art of being present, individuals can lead more fulfilling and balanced lives.

Mindful Awareness In Everyday Life

Mindful awareness is a practice that encourages individuals to be fully present in their daily lives, even during the most routine activities. It involves a conscious and non-judgmental observation of thoughts, emotions, and sensations as they arise. Here's how mindful awareness can be integrated into everyday life:

Morning Routine: Begin the day with mindful awareness. Instead of rushing through your morning routine, take the time to savor each moment. Feel the warmth of the water during your shower, savor the taste of your breakfast, and appreciate the morning sunlight.

Mindful Breathing: Throughout the day, take moments to focus on your breath. Pay attention to the rise and fall of your chest or the sensation of the breath passing through your nostrils. This practice can be done while waiting in line, during a short break, or in between tasks.

Eating Mindfully: When you eat, engage your senses fully. Notice the colors, textures, and flavors of your food. Chew slowly and savor each bite. This not only enhances the enjoyment of your meal but also aids in digestion.

Walking Meditation: Walking can be a mindful activity. Pay attention to each step, the feeling of your feet touching the ground, and the sensation of movement. This can be done during a stroll in the park or even while walking from one room to another.

Technology Breaks: In the age of constant digital connectivity, take mindful breaks from screens. Put away your phone and computer for a few minutes and simply observe your surroundings. Listen to the sounds, feel the air, and appreciate the moment.

Observing Emotions: When you experience emotions, whether positive or negative, observe them without judgment. Recognize the feelings as they arise, and allow yourself to feel them without trying to change or suppress them.

Gratitude Practice: Regularly take a moment to reflect on the things you're grateful for. This practice fosters a sense of appreciation for the present moment and the positive aspects of your life.

Mindful Listening: When in conversation with others, practice mindful listening. Instead of formulating your response while the other person is speaking, truly hear their words and try to understand their perspective.

Single-Tasking: In a world that often glorifies multitasking, try single-tasking instead. Focus on one task at a time, giving it your full attention. This not only increases efficiency but also allows for a deeper connection to the task at hand.

Evening Reflection: At the end of the day, reflect on your experiences with a sense of mindfulness. What moments brought you joy, and what challenges did you face? This practice helps you process your day and prepare for a restful night.

Breathing Space: During stressful moments, create a "breathing space." Take a few deep breaths and bring your awareness to the sensations in your body. This can help you respond to stressors with greater calm and clarity.

Mindful Activities: Engage in activities you love with mindfulness. Whether it's gardening, playing a musical instrument, or painting, immerse yourself fully in the activity, appreciating the sensory experience it offers.

Observing Nature: Spend time in nature with a sense of mindful awareness. Observe the beauty of the natural world, whether it's the rustling leaves of a tree, the sound of a flowing stream, or the colors of a sunset.

Mindful awareness in everyday life is about living in the present moment, fully engaged with your experiences. It can enhance the quality of your life, reduce stress, and promote a deeper sense of well-being. Through these practices, you can cultivate a profound connection to the world around you and your own inner self.

Exercises To Enhance Present-Moment Living

Cultivating present-moment living requires practice and intention. Here are some exercises to enhance your ability to stay in the present moment:

Mindful Breathing: Sit or lie down in a comfortable position. Close your eyes and take a few deep breaths. Then, shift your attention to your natural breath. Observe the sensation of your breath as it enters and leaves your body. When your mind wanders, gently bring your focus back to your breath.

Body Scan: Find a quiet space and lie down. Starting from your toes, bring your awareness to each part of your body, moving upwards. Notice any sensations, tension, or discomfort. Breathe into those areas, allowing them to relax. This exercise helps you connect with your body and release physical tension.

Five Senses Check-In: Pause and take a moment to engage each of your five senses. What can you see, hear, smell, taste, and touch right now? This exercise instantly grounds you in the present moment by focusing on sensory experiences.

Mindful Eating: Choose a piece of food, such as a raisin or a small piece of chocolate. Before eating it, examine it closely, noticing its texture and color. As you take a bite, savor the taste and chew slowly, paying attention to the flavors and sensations in your mouth.

Walking Meditation: Take a walk with mindful awareness. Focus on each step as it connects with the ground. Feel the rise and fall of your feet, the movement of your legs, and the sensation of walking. Engage all your senses in the act of walking.

Breathing Space: When you feel stressed or overwhelmed, create a breathing space. Find a quiet spot and take a few deep breaths. Bring your attention to your breath and observe it for a minute or two. This exercise helps you regain a sense of calm in the midst of chaos.

Observing Emotions: When an emotion arises, be it joy, anger, or sadness, pause to observe it without judgment. Name the emotion and feel it fully without trying to change it. This exercise encourages emotional self-awareness.

Nature Connection: Spend time in nature. Whether you're in a park or the wilderness, be fully present in the natural surroundings. Observe the beauty of the environment, listen to the sounds of nature, and feel the earth beneath your feet.

Mindful Appreciation: Choose an object or person and contemplate what you appreciate about it. It could be a loved one, a pet, a favorite book, or a work of art. Reflect on the positive aspects and feelings it evokes.

Single-Tasking: Practice doing one task at a time with full attention. Whether it's washing dishes, reading a book, or working on a project, immerse yourself in the activity without distractions or the urge to multitask.

Gratitude Journal: Keep a gratitude journal where you write down things you're grateful for each day. This exercise encourages you to focus on positive aspects of your life and appreciate them.

Mindful Listening: When engaged in a conversation, practice

active listening. Give the speaker your full attention without formulating responses in your mind. Be present in the moment, hearing and understanding what is being communicated.

Daily Reflection: At the end of the day, reflect on your experiences with a sense of mindfulness. What moments brought you joy, and what challenges did you face? This practice helps you process your day and prepare for a restful night.

By incorporating these exercises into your daily life, you can strengthen your ability to live in the present moment. Over time, mindful living becomes a natural and enriching way to experience the world around you.

CHAPTER 5: THE INNER JOURNEY

Exploring Self-Discovery And Inner Peace

Self-discovery is a transformative journey that leads to inner peace, personal growth, and a deeper understanding of oneself. To embark on this journey, consider the following steps and practices:

Self-Reflection: Set aside quiet time for self-reflection. Journal your thoughts, emotions, and experiences. This practice helps you gain insight into your inner world and identify patterns in your thoughts and behavior.

Mindfulness Meditation: Engage in mindfulness meditation to quiet your mind and observe your thoughts without judgment. This practice fosters self-awareness and a sense of inner calm.

Exploring Passions: Discover your passions and interests by trying new activities and hobbies. Exploring what genuinely excites you can lead to a deeper connection with your true self.

Self-Compassion: Cultivate self-compassion by treating yourself with the same kindness and understanding you offer to others. Be gentle with your imperfections and embrace self-acceptance.

Uncovering Core Values: Identify your core values and principles. Understanding what truly matters to you can guide your decisions and actions, promoting a sense of alignment with your authentic self.

Seeking Feedback: Ask for feedback from trusted friends and family. They can provide valuable insights into your strengths and areas for growth, helping you on your path to self-discovery.

Exploring Spirituality: Explore spirituality or connect with your existing spiritual beliefs. Many find a sense of inner peace and purpose through spiritual practices.

Embracing Solitude: Spend time alone in solitude. Solitude allows you to connect with your inner thoughts and feelings, fostering self-discovery and reflection.

Letting Go of the Past: Release any emotional baggage from the past. Forgiving yourself and others is a crucial step toward finding inner peace and self-acceptance.

Living in the Present: Embrace the present moment by practicing mindfulness. Focus on the here and now, letting go of worries about the future and regrets from the past.

Setting Boundaries: Establish healthy boundaries in your relationships and daily life. Protect your well-being by honoring your limits and priorities.

Gratitude and Positive Thinking: Cultivate gratitude by recognizing the positive aspects of your life. Shifting your focus toward appreciation promotes a sense of inner peace and contentment.

Seeking Guidance: Consider seeking guidance from a therapist, coach, or mentor who can provide support and insights as you navigate your path of self-discovery.

Challenging Comfort Zones: Step out of your comfort zones and face new challenges. Growth often occurs when you embrace discomfort and expand your horizons.

Self-Care Practices: Prioritize self-care through practices like exercise, a balanced diet, adequate sleep, and stress management. A healthy body can lead to a healthier mind.

Mind-Body Practices: Engage in mind-body practices like yoga, tai chi, or qigong to harmonize the connection between your mental and physical well-being.

Seeking Inner Peace: The journey of self-discovery ultimately leads to inner peace. Embrace inner peace as a state of mind where you find contentment, acceptance, and serenity.

Self-discovery is an ongoing process that can bring you closer to your authentic self and lead to a profound sense of inner peace and fulfillment. Embrace these practices to explore your inner world and embark on a transformative journey of self-discovery.

Practices For Self-Acceptance And Self-Compassion

Self-acceptance and self-compassion are vital components of a healthy and fulfilling life. Here are practices to cultivate these qualities:

Positive Affirmations: Replace self-criticism with positive self-affirmations. Speak kindly to yourself and challenge negative thoughts with uplifting statements.

Mindful Self-Compassion: Practice self-compassion meditation, focusing on your suffering with a kind and non-judgmental attitude. Treat yourself as you would a dear friend in times of difficulty.

Self-Reflection: Take time for self-reflection to understand your values, strengths, and areas for growth. Accept that imperfections are a part of being human.

Letting Go of Perfection: Embrace your imperfections and let go of the need for perfection. Understand that mistakes and flaws are opportunities for learning and growth.

Gratitude Journal: Maintain a gratitude journal where you list things you appreciate about yourself and your life. Practicing gratitude reinforces self-acceptance.

Celebrate Achievements: Acknowledge and celebrate your accomplishments, no matter how small they may seem. Recognizing your successes boosts self-esteem.

Healthy Self-Talk: Monitor your self-talk and reframe negative thoughts. Treat yourself with kindness and understanding, especially during challenging times.

Self-Care Rituals: Prioritize self-care rituals, whether it's exercise, meditation, spa days, or hobbies. Nurturing yourself demonstrates self-compassion.

Seek Support: Reach out to a therapist or support group for assistance with self-acceptance and self-compassion. Professional guidance can be invaluable.

Forgiveness: Forgive yourself for past mistakes and let go of grudges. Holding onto guilt or resentment hinders self-compassion and acceptance.

Boundaries: Set healthy boundaries in your relationships. Protect your well-being and communicate your needs with respect and assertiveness.

Mindful Breathing: During moments of self-doubt or criticism, practice mindful breathing. Breathe deeply, focusing on the present moment, and let go of self-judgment.

Self-Compassionate Letter: Write a letter to yourself as if you were writing to a dear friend who's experiencing the same struggles. Offer words of understanding and support.

Humanize Imperfections: Understand that everyone has flaws and makes mistakes. Embrace your humanity and recognize that these imperfections are part of your unique journey.

Self-Love Rituals: Incorporate self-love rituals, such as self-massage, self-hugging, or self-soothing gestures, to express love and care for yourself.

Visualization: Visualize yourself as a loving and compassionate friend. Imagine how this friend would treat you during challenging times, and practice self-compassion accordingly.

Mindful Eating: Practice mindful eating by savoring your meals and treating your body with nourishing foods. Cultivating a positive relationship with your body is a form of self-acceptance.

Staying Present: Engage in mindfulness exercises to stay present in the moment. Redirect your focus away from self-criticism and toward self-compassion.

Small Acts of Kindness: Perform small acts of kindness for yourself regularly. Whether it's a relaxing bath, a walk in nature, or a favorite treat, these gestures foster self-compassion.

Daily Gratitude: Each day, express gratitude for the unique qualities and experiences that make you who you are. Recognize the value you bring to the world.

By incorporating these practices into your life, you can cultivate a deep sense of self-acceptance and self-compassion. These qualities are essential for building a foundation of self-esteem, resilience, and well-being.

Navigating The Challenges Of The Inner Journey

The path of self-discovery and inner peace is not always smooth, and challenges are an integral part of the journey. Here's how to navigate these challenges effectively:

Self-Doubt: When self-doubt arises, remind yourself of your strengths and past accomplishments. Embrace uncertainty as an opportunity for growth.

Overcoming Fear: Face your fears head-on. Understand that fear often signifies areas where personal growth and transformation can occur. Take small steps to confront your fears.

Resisting Change: Change can be uncomfortable, even when it's positive. Embrace change as a natural part of life and focus on the potential benefits it may bring.

Dealing with Uncertainty: Uncertainty is a constant in life. Accept that not everything can be controlled or predicted. Cultivate resilience and adaptability to face uncertainty with grace.

Negative Self-Talk: Challenge negative self-talk and limiting beliefs. Replace them with positive affirmations and constructive self-dialogue. Seek support from a therapist or counselor if needed.

Balancing Self-Care: Self-discovery often involves introspection and emotional exploration. Balance this with self-care practices that nurture your mental and emotional well-being.

Patience and Persistence: Be patient with yourself, as self-discovery is an ongoing journey. It may take time to find inner peace and understand yourself fully. Stay persistent and committed to the path.

Facing Past Trauma: Addressing past trauma can be challenging. Seek professional support to guide you through the healing process. Healing is a brave and transformative step.

Finding Inner Peace: Inner peace is not a constant state but rather a practice. When you feel inner turmoil, engage in mindfulness, meditation, or other calming activities to restore peace.

Maintaining Boundaries: Set boundaries in relationships to protect your energy and well-being. Communicate your needs clearly and assertively to maintain a healthy balance.

Comparison and Judgement: Avoid comparing yourself to others or harsh self-judgment. Embrace your unique path and experiences, and celebrate your individuality.

Forgiveness: Forgiving yourself and others can be challenging but is essential for inner peace. Practice forgiveness to release emotional burdens and find closure.

Adapting to Change: Life is constantly evolving, and your self-discovery journey may lead you in new directions. Embrace change with an open heart, knowing that it can bring growth.

Staying Present: When challenges overwhelm you, practice staying present in the moment. Mindfulness and deep breathing can help you remain centered and focused.

Accepting Setbacks: Understand that setbacks are a natural part of any journey. When setbacks occur, use them as opportunities to learn and grow.

Self-Compassion: Be gentle with yourself during challenging times. Offer self-compassion and treat yourself as you would a dear friend.

Seeking Support: Reach out to a support network, therapist, or counselor when challenges become overwhelming. Professional guidance can provide valuable insights and strategies.

Maintaining Perspective: Keep the bigger picture in mind. Challenges are often stepping stones to personal growth and self-awareness.

Resisting External Pressure: Tune out external pressures and expectations. Your inner journey is unique, and you have the freedom to explore it at your own pace.

Embracing Vulnerability: Embrace vulnerability as a source of strength. Sharing your challenges and experiences with others can create connections and support your inner journey.

Remember that challenges are an integral part of the inner journey, and they can lead to profound personal growth and transformation. Embrace them as opportunities for self-discovery and the path to lasting inner peace.

CHAPTER6: MINDFUL LIVING IN A FAST-PACED WORLD

Mindfulness Amidst Chaos

In times of chaos and upheaval, practicing mindfulness can be a powerful tool for maintaining inner calm and clarity. Here's how to cultivate mindfulness amidst chaos:

Breathe Mindfully: Take slow, deep breaths to center yourself. Focus on your breath, inhaling and exhaling consciously. This simple practice can help anchor you in the present moment.

Acknowledge Your Emotions: Recognize and accept your emotions without judgment. It's natural to feel a range of emotions during chaotic times. Observing them without resistance can help you manage them more effectively.

Stay Present: Remind yourself to stay present in the moment. Avoid ruminating on the past or worrying about the future. Engage fully in what you are doing at the present moment.

Mindful Observation: Take a moment to observe your surroundings. Notice the colors, shapes, and textures of objects. Listen to the sounds around you. Grounding yourself in sensory experiences can be calming.

Let Go of Control: Chaos often arises from a lack of control. Practice letting go of the need to control every situation. Embrace uncertainty and trust in your ability to adapt.

Practice Gratitude: Even in chaotic times, find things to be grateful for. Maintaining a gratitude practice can shift your focus toward the positive aspects of your life.

Limit Information Overload: In the age of information, it's easy to become overwhelmed by news and updates. Set boundaries on the amount of information you consume and choose reliable sources.

Mindful Self-Care: Prioritize self-care, even in chaotic moments. Engage in activities that bring you joy and relaxation, whether it's reading, listening to music, or taking a warm bath.

Mindful Eating: When you eat, do so mindfully. Savor the flavors, textures, and aromas of your food. Eating with mindfulness can be a nourishing and calming experience.

Connect with Others: Reach out to friends and loved ones for support and connection. Sharing your thoughts and feelings can alleviate stress and provide emotional relief.

Avoid Multitasking: Focus on one task at a time. Multitasking can add to feelings of chaos and overwhelm. Completing one task mindfully before moving on to the next can enhance efficiency and peace of mind.

Mindful Listening: When in conversation, practice active listening. Give your full attention to the speaker, validating their emotions and perspectives. This fosters deeper connections.

Set Boundaries: Establish boundaries with respect to your time, energy, and relationships. Protect your well-being by clearly communicating your limits.

Mindful Movement: Engage in mindful movement practices like yoga, tai chi, or qigong. These activities promote a sense of balance, both physically and mentally.

Practice Patience: Cultivate patience with yourself and others. Chaos can create stress and tension, and patience is a valuable tool for diffusing challenging situations.

Release Judgment: Let go of judgment, both of yourself and others. Practice self-compassion and offer understanding to those around you. Accept that everyone is navigating chaos in their own way.

Gratitude for Lessons: View chaotic times as opportunities for growth and learning. Embrace the lessons that arise from adversity.

Prioritize Well-Being: Make well-being a priority. Engage in practices that promote physical, mental, and emotional health. A balanced and healthy lifestyle can help you withstand chaos more effectively.

Cultivating mindfulness amidst chaos is a skill that can enhance your resilience and inner peace. It allows you to navigate challenging times with grace and a sense of centeredness.

Strategies For Integrating Mindfulness Into A Busy Life

In the midst of a hectic and busy life, incorporating mindfulness can be transformative. Here are strategies to seamlessly integrate mindfulness into your daily routine:

Mindful Morning Routine: Begin your day with intention. Dedicate a few minutes for mindful breathing, stretching, or a short meditation to set a positive tone for the day.

Mindful Commute: If you commute, use this time for mindfulness. Focus on your breath, the scenery, or listen to calming music. Transform a daily chore into a mindfulness practice.

Mindful Eating: During meals, practice mindful eating. Pay attention to the colors, textures, and flavors of your food. Chew slowly and savor each bite, fully engaging with the experience.

Mindful Walking: When you walk from one place to another, do so mindfully. Feel the ground beneath your feet, notice your surroundings, and be present in your steps.

Micro-Mindfulness Breaks: Take short breaks during the day to reset. Close your eyes, take a few deep breaths, and refocus your attention. These micro-mindfulness breaks can enhance productivity and reduce stress.

Technology Boundaries: Set boundaries with technology. Designate tech-free zones or times to unplug and reconnect with the present moment.

Mindful Conversations: Practice mindful listening during conversations. Be fully present with the speaker, offering your complete attention and empathy.

Mindful Waiting: Utilize waiting periods, whether in line or at appointments, for mindfulness. Engage in deep breathing or observe your surroundings without distraction.

Mindful Posture: Be mindful of your posture throughout the day. Sit and stand with intention, focusing on your alignment and how it feels in your body.

Mindful Breathing: Return to your breath as an anchor. Take a few moments to breathe mindfully, whether at your desk, in your car, or during transitions between tasks.

Mindful Stress Response: When stress arises, pause and breathe mindfully before reacting. This practice can help you respond to stressors with greater composure.

Mindful Gratitude: Express gratitude throughout the day. Reflect on the things you're thankful for, no matter how small. This practice can shift your focus to positivity.

Mindful Decluttering: Engage in mindful decluttering and organization. Approach these tasks with presence and awareness, letting go of what no longer serves you.

Mindful Reflection: Before bed, spend a few minutes in mindful reflection. Review your day, acknowledging your achievements and areas for improvement.

Mindful Technology Use: Consciously use technology for mindfulness. There are various apps and resources that offer guided meditation and mindfulness exercises. Incorporate them into your digital routine.

Mindful Breathing Exercises: Learn and practice specific mindful breathing exercises that you can use as tools throughout your day, such as the 4-7-8 breath or box breathing.

Mindful Gratitude Journal: Keep a gratitude journal to jot down things you're thankful for. Take a moment to write in it daily or weekly.

Mindful Reminders: Set reminders on your phone or computer to pause and breathe mindfully, ensuring you infuse mindfulness into your busy schedule.

Mindful Transition Rituals: Create mindful transition rituals between different tasks or roles. These rituals can signal a shift in focus and help you stay present.

Mindful Sleep: Practice a bedtime mindfulness routine to relax and prepare for sleep. It can include meditation, gentle stretching, or calming breathing exercises.

By implementing these strategies, you can seamlessly integrate mindfulness into your busy life, enhancing your well-being and overall sense of balance amidst a hectic schedule.

Balancing Technology And Mindfulness

In today's digital age, balancing technology with mindfulness is essential for maintaining mental and emotional well-being. Here are strategies to find equilibrium in a tech-savvy world:

Set Tech Boundaries: Establish clear boundaries for technology use. Designate tech-free times or zones, such as during meals, before bed, or in specific rooms of your home.

Mindful Notifications: Customize your notifications to minimize distractions. Allow only essential notifications and turn off non-essential ones to reduce constant interruptions.

Digital Detox: Regularly disconnect from technology. Schedule tech-free days or weekends to unwind and reconnect with the physical world.

Tech-Free Mornings: Begin your day without immediately checking your phone or computer. Use the morning for mindful practices like meditation, journaling, or enjoying breakfast without screens.

Mindful Social Media: Practice mindful use of social media. Be conscious of the time you spend on platforms, and curate your online experience by following accounts that inspire and uplift you.

Digital Sabbaticals: Take extended breaks from technology. Whether it's a weeklong vacation or a weekend retreat, periodically unplug to recharge.

Mindful Email Management: Set specific times to check and respond to emails. Avoid checking your email constantly, which can be overwhelming and distracting.

Tech-Free Hobbies: Cultivate hobbies that don't involve screens. Engage in activities like painting, gardening, or playing a musical instrument to balance screen time.

Screen-Free Meals: Make mealtime a screen-free zone. Focus on the food, taste, and company of loved ones, enhancing the dining experience.

Mindful Tech Choices: Be mindful of the apps and websites you use. Delete or limit access to those that contribute to stress or excessive screen time.

Tech-Free Breaks: Take short tech breaks during the day. Step away from screens, stretch, and practice mindfulness to refresh your mind and reduce eye strain.

Mindful Gaming: If you're a gamer, be intentional about your gaming time. Play mindfully and avoid overindulgence, especially late at night.

Digital Awareness: Cultivate awareness of your digital behavior.

Regularly reflect on how technology impacts your life, emotions, and relationships.

Tech-Enhanced Mindfulness: Use technology to support your mindfulness practice. There are apps and online resources that offer guided meditations and mindfulness exercises.

Mindful Social Connections: Nurture authentic social connections by engaging in meaningful conversations and in-person interactions. Use technology to enhance, not replace, human connections.

Screen Sleep Ritual: Create a screen sleep ritual by turning off screens at least an hour before bedtime. Engage in calming activities like reading, stretching, or gentle yoga.

Digital Clutter: Declutter your digital life by organizing files, emails, and apps. A clean digital environment can promote mental clarity.

Mindful Screen Time: When using technology, be present and attentive. Avoid mindless scrolling and multitasking, and focus on the task at hand.

Tech-Free Retreats: Consider attending tech-free retreats or workshops to deepen your mindfulness practice and regain balance.

Tech and Nature: Spend time in nature without screens. Disconnect from technology and immerse yourself in the beauty and serenity of the natural world.

Balancing technology and mindfulness is an ongoing journey. By implementing these strategies, you can harness the benefits of technology while nurturing your mental, emotional, and spiritual well-being.

CHAPTER 7: MINDFUL RELATIONSHIPS

Building Mindful Connections With Others

Creating mindful connections with people is a profound way to enhance relationships and foster emotional well-being. Here's how to build meaningful, mindful connections with others:

Present Listening: When engaged in conversation, practice active listening. Be fully present with the speaker, giving them your undivided attention. Avoid interrupting or formulating responses while they're speaking.

Empathy: Cultivate empathy by trying to understand the emotions and perspectives of others. Put yourself in their shoes and acknowledge their feelings, even if you don't share the same experiences.

Non-judgment: Suspend judgment and refrain from making assumptions about others. Embrace the idea that everyone has their unique life journey and experiences.

Open Communication: Encourage open and honest communication. Create a safe space for people to express themselves without fear of criticism or rejection.

Kindness: Treat others with kindness and compassion. Small acts of kindness, whether a smile or a thoughtful gesture, can strengthen connections.

Mindful Presence: Be fully present when spending time with others. Avoid distractions like phones or other devices, and focus on the person in front of you.

Shared Activities: Engage in shared activities that promote mindfulness, such as meditating together, practicing yoga, or going for a mindful walk. These activities can deepen connections.

Quality Time: Allocate quality time for your relationships. Dedicate time for meaningful interactions, whether it's a heartfelt conversation or simply enjoying each other's company.

Forgiveness: Practice forgiveness and let go of grudges or past grievances. Holding onto resentment can hinder connections.

Authenticity: Be authentic and true to yourself in your interactions. Authenticity fosters genuine connections based on trust and openness.

Express Gratitude: Regularly express gratitude for the people in your life. Let them know you appreciate and value their presence.

Supportive Relationships: Cultivate relationships that provide emotional support and encouragement. Surround yourself with people who uplift and inspire you.

Boundaries: Set healthy boundaries in your relationships. Clearly communicate your needs and respect the boundaries of others to maintain balance and mutual respect.

Conflict Resolution: Address conflicts mindfully and constructively. Approach disagreements with understanding and a willingness to find common ground.

Mindful Touch: Physical touch, like hugs or handshakes, can convey mindfulness and warmth. Use touch as a way to connect with others on a deeper level.

Gratitude Journal: Keep a gratitude journal specifically for the people in your life. Reflect on the positive impact they've had and the qualities you admire in them.

Supportive Conversations: Engage in supportive conversations by asking open-ended questions and actively participating in the dialogue. Encourage the sharing of thoughts and feelings.

Celebrate Milestones: Celebrate important milestones and achievements of the people in your life. Acknowledging their successes strengthens connections.

Mindful Acknowledgment: Take a moment to mindfully acknowledge the presence and well-being of others. Wish them health, happiness, and peace in your thoughts or words.

Deepening Connections: Invest in deepening connections with those who matter most to you. Dedicate time and effort to nurture these relationships.

Building mindful connections with others not only enriches your life but also contributes to the well-being and happiness of those around you. These connections are a source of support, love, and shared experiences.

Communication And Conflict Resolution

Active Listening: Practice active listening by giving your full attention to the speaker. Avoid interrupting and aim to understand their perspective before responding.

Clear and Concise: Communicate your thoughts clearly and concisely. Use simple language to avoid misunderstandings.

Non-Verbal Cues: Pay attention to non-verbal cues, such as body language and facial expressions, to gain insights into the speaker's emotions and intentions.

Empathy: Cultivate empathy by trying to understand the other person's feelings and point of view. Acknowledge their emotions.

Open-Ended Questions: Encourage open dialogue by asking open-ended questions that invite thoughtful responses and promote discussion.

I-Statements: Use "I" statements to express your feelings and needs, such as "I feel" or "I need." This approach is less confrontational and encourages understanding.

Tone of Voice: Be mindful of your tone of voice. Use a calm and respectful tone, even when discussing sensitive topics.

Pause and Reflect: Take a moment to pause and reflect before responding, especially in heated discussions. This can prevent impulsive reactions.

Avoid Assumptions: Refrain from making assumptions about the other person's thoughts or intentions. Clarify any uncertainties by asking for clarification.

Respect Boundaries: Respect personal boundaries, both in your communication and in the topics you discuss. Ensure that the other person is comfortable with the conversation.

Conflict Resolution:

Address Issues Promptly: Don't let conflicts fester. Address issues promptly to prevent them from escalating.

Use "I" Statements: When discussing conflicts, express your feelings and needs using "I" statements to avoid blame and defensiveness.

Active Problem-Solving: Collaboratively work on finding solutions to conflicts. Encourage open dialogue to identify common ground and resolutions.

Stay Calm: Keep your emotions in check during conflicts. Emotional reactions can hinder effective resolution.

Listen Actively: In conflict discussions, ensure that both parties have the opportunity to express their perspectives and concerns. Listen actively to each other.

Find Compromises: Seek compromises that are acceptable to both parties. Be open to negotiation and finding middle ground.

Take Breaks: If tensions rise during a conflict discussion, it's acceptable to take a break to cool off and regain composure before continuing the conversation.

Avoid Blame: Focus on the issue at hand rather than assigning blame. Blame can lead to defensiveness and hinder resolution.

Accept Differences: Recognize that differences in opinions and perspectives are natural. Accept these differences without judgment.

Seek Mediation: In cases where conflicts are particularly challenging, consider seeking mediation from a neutral third party, such as a counselor or mediator.

Closure and Forgiveness: Once a conflict is resolved, seek closure and forgiveness. Let go of lingering negative feelings to restore harmony.

Learn from Conflicts: View conflicts as opportunities for personal and relational growth. Learn from each conflict to prevent similar issues in the future.

Effective communication and conflict resolution contribute to healthier and more fulfilling relationships. These skills promote understanding, empathy, and cooperation, fostering greater harmony in personal and professional connections.

Mindfulness In Love And Relationships

Mindfulness can significantly enhance love and relationships by fostering emotional presence and connection. Here are ways to incorporate mindfulness into your romantic life:

Present Together Time: When spending time with your partner, be fully present. Put away distractions and savor the moments you share.

Mindful Listening: Practice active listening during conversations. Give your partner your full attention, and genuinely empathize with their emotions and experiences.

Non-Judgment: Suspend judgment in your interactions. Accept your partner as they are, and let go of preconceived notions or expectations.

Gratitude: Express gratitude for your partner and the positive aspects of your relationship. Regularly acknowledge the love and joy they bring to your life.

Loving-Kindness Meditation: Engage in loving-kindness meditation to cultivate feelings of love, compassion, and goodwill towards your partner and yourself.

Mindful Communication: Communicate mindfully by choosing words thoughtfully and speaking with kindness and respect.

Conflict Resolution: When conflicts arise, approach them mindfully. Engage in calm, rational discussions and seek mutually satisfying resolutions.

Quality Time: Prioritize quality time together. Engage in activities that nurture your connection, whether it's a date night, a romantic getaway, or a quiet evening at home.

Mindful Affection: When you express affection, do so with presence. Hug, kiss, or hold hands mindfully, appreciating the physical and emotional connection.

Mindful Sexuality: In intimate moments, be fully present and attuned to your partner's desires and needs. Focus on the emotional and physical aspects of the experience.

Forgiveness: Practice forgiveness and let go of past grievances. Holding onto grudges can hinder the growth of love and intimacy.

Intention Setting: Set loving intentions for your relationship. Visualize the kind of loving and harmonious partnership you want to create.

Affirmations: Use affirmations to reinforce love and positivity in your relationship. Share loving affirmations with your partner.

Mindful Meals: When dining together, mindfully savor the food and each other's company. Use this time to connect and bond.

Relationship Mindfulness Ritual: Create a relationship mindfulness ritual. It could be a daily check-in or a weekly reflection on your relationship's progress.

Spontaneity: Embrace spontaneity by surprising your partner with gestures of love and affection. Small surprises can keep the relationship fresh and exciting.

Mindful Separation: When you're apart, maintain a sense of connection through mindful communication and expressions of affection.

Reflect on Love: Periodically reflect on the love and connection you share. This can strengthen your appreciation for each other.

Couples Mindfulness Classes: Consider taking couples mindfulness classes or workshops to deepen your practice together.

Renewal Rituals: Establish renewal rituals, such as anniversaries, to reaffirm your commitment and love for each other.

Mindfulness in love and relationships promotes deeper emotional bonds, understanding, and joy. By practicing these strategies, you can create a more loving and harmonious partnership.

CHAPTER 8: MINDFULNESS AND MENTAL HEALTH

Mindfulness For Stress Reduction

Mindfulness is a powerful tool for reducing stress and enhancing overall well-being. Here's how to incorporate mindfulness into your life to effectively manage and reduce stress:

Mindful Breathing: Practice mindful breathing by taking deep, intentional breaths. Focus on your breath's rhythm, and use it as an anchor to the present moment.

Body Scan Meditation: Engage in body scan meditations to tune into physical sensations and release tension. Begin at your head and work your way down to your toes, relaxing each body part.

Mindful Eating: Savor your meals mindfully. Pay attention to the colors, textures, and flavors of your food. Chew slowly and fully engage in the act of eating.

Mindful Walking: Take mindful walks, paying attention to the movement of your body and the sensations in your surroundings.

Notice the rhythm of your steps and the sounds of nature.

Mindful Relaxation: Dedicate time to mindful relaxation. Whether it's through meditation, yoga, or deep breathing exercises, relax with intention to release stress.

Daily Gratitude: Cultivate gratitude by reflecting on the things you're thankful for each day. This practice shifts your focus to positivity and reduces stress.

Acceptance and Non-Judgment: Practice non-judgment and acceptance of your thoughts and emotions. Understand that it's natural to have stress, and don't judge yourself for feeling it.

Mindful Work Breaks: Take short mindfulness breaks during your workday. Step away from your tasks, close your eyes, and take a few deep breaths to reset and refocus.

Mindful Technology Use: Be mindful of your technology use. Set boundaries for screen time to prevent information overload and constant connectivity stress.

Mindful Communication: Use mindful communication in your interactions. Listen actively and respond thoughtfully, promoting clear and empathetic conversations.

Mindful Time Management: Manage your time mindfully. Prioritize tasks, and avoid overcommitting to prevent stress from overwhelming your schedule.

Nature Connection: Spend time in nature to recharge. Nature's tranquility and beauty can be a natural stress reducer.

Mindful Visualization: Use visualization techniques to create a mental sanctuary where you can escape stress. Imagine a calm, peaceful place where you can retreat mentally.

Mindful Self-Compassion: Be kind and compassionate to yourself. Acknowledge your stress without self-criticism, and treat yourself with the same care you'd offer a friend.

Mindful Sleep: Develop a mindful bedtime routine to ensure restful sleep. Disconnect from screens, engage in calming activities, and practice relaxation techniques before bed.

Mindful Breakdown of Tasks: When tackling tasks, break them down into smaller, manageable steps. This approach reduces the stress of overwhelming projects.

Mindful Acceptance of Imperfection: Accept that perfection isn't attainable. Embrace your imperfections and learn to appreciate yourself as you are.

Mindful Journaling: Maintain a mindfulness journal to record your thoughts, emotions, and stress triggers. This self-awareness can help you manage stress more effectively.

Mindful Breathing Techniques: Learn and practice specific mindful breathing techniques, such as the 4-7-8 breath or box breathing, to reduce stress and anxiety.

Mindful Support Network: Seek support from friends, family, or support groups when stress becomes overwhelming. Share your feelings and challenges mindfully.

By incorporating mindfulness into your daily life, you can reduce stress, enhance your coping mechanisms, and find a greater sense of calm and balance, even in the face of life's challenges.

Mindfulness-Based Approaches To Anxiety And

Depression

Mindfulness-based approaches offer effective strategies for managing and alleviating symptoms of anxiety and depression. Here are ways to incorporate mindfulness into your life to address these mental health challenges:

Mindful Awareness:

Emotional Acceptance: Embrace your emotions without judgment. Mindfulness encourages you to acknowledge your feelings without self-criticism.

Present-Moment Focus: Shift your attention to the present moment. Mindfulness practices, such as deep breathing or body scans, can ground you in the "here and now."

Thought Observation: Observe your thoughts objectively. Recognize that thoughts are transient and not necessarily reflective of reality.

Cultivate Self-Compassion: Practice self-compassion by treating yourself with the same kindness and understanding you'd offer a friend in distress.

Mindful Body Awareness: Pay attention to bodily sensations associated with anxiety and depression. Understanding these physical cues can help manage emotional symptoms.

Mindful Meditation and Relaxation:

Breathing Exercises: Engage in mindful breathing exercises to calm your mind and reduce anxiety. Techniques like diaphragmatic breathing can be particularly beneficial.

Guided Meditations: Follow guided mindfulness meditations,

which are widely available online and through apps. These meditations can help alleviate symptoms and promote relaxation.

Progressive Muscle Relaxation: Practice progressive muscle relaxation to release physical tension associated with anxiety and depression.

Mindful Yoga: Incorporate mindful yoga into your routine. It combines physical activity with mindfulness, promoting relaxation and stress reduction.

Mindful Coping Strategies:

Mindful Journaling: Keep a mindfulness journal to document your thoughts, feelings, and triggers. This self-awareness can help identify patterns and manage emotions.

Stress Reduction Techniques: Explore various stress reduction techniques like mindful coloring, nature walks, or engaging in creative activities.

Mindful Sleep Practices: Develop a mindful sleep routine to improve the quality of your rest. This can help alleviate depressive symptoms related to sleep disturbances.

Mindfulness-Based Cognitive Therapy (MBCT):

MBCT Programs: Consider participating in structured MBCT programs, which combine cognitive therapy with mindfulness practices to prevent relapse in depression and manage anxiety.

Mindful Focus on Thought Patterns: Use MBCT to explore and challenge negative thought patterns and cultivate more adaptive thinking.

Mindful Self-Compassion:

Self-Compassion Exercises: Practice self-compassion exercises to foster kindness towards yourself, even when experiencing challenging emotions.
Professional Guidance:

Mindfulness-Based Therapy: Seek the guidance of a mental health professional experienced in mindfulness-based therapies, such as Mindfulness-Based Stress Reduction (MBSR) or MBCT.

Individual Counseling: Consider individual counseling or therapy with a focus on mindfulness to address specific anxiety and depression symptoms.

Group Support: Join mindfulness-based support groups or workshops. These group settings can provide a sense of community and shared experiences.

Medication and Mindfulness: If prescribed medication, continue it as directed by a healthcare professional while simultaneously integrating mindfulness practices into your routine.

Open Communication: Maintain open communication with your healthcare provider regarding your mindfulness journey and its impact on your mental health.

Mindfulness-based approaches empower individuals to develop healthier coping mechanisms for anxiety and depression. By embracing mindfulness, you can cultivate resilience and find relief from these challenging conditions.

Techniques For Emotional Resilience

Emotional resilience is the ability to bounce back from adversity, adapt to change, and maintain mental and emotional well-being. Here are techniques to build and strengthen emotional resilience:

1. Mindfulness and Self-Awareness:

Practice mindfulness to stay present and aware of your emotions.
Reflect on your emotional responses without judgment.
Keep a journal to track your feelings and thought patterns.
2. Emotional Regulation:

Develop strategies to manage intense emotions, such as deep breathing or progressive muscle relaxation.
Use positive self-talk to reframe negative thoughts and emotions.
Visualize calming and soothing images during stressful moments.
3. Social Support:

Build and nurture a support network of friends and family.
Seek out support groups or counseling when facing difficult challenges.
Share your feelings and concerns with someone you trust.
4. Problem-Solving:

Break problems into manageable steps to make them less overwhelming.
Seek solutions and take action to address issues rather than dwelling on them.
Learn to adapt and adjust when faced with unexpected obstacles.
5. Resilience-Building Activities:

Engage in physical activity to release stress and boost endorphins.
Pursue hobbies and interests that bring joy and a sense of accomplishment.
Set achievable goals to foster a sense of purpose.
6. Optimism and Positivity:

Cultivate a positive outlook and focus on silver linings in challenging situations.
Practice gratitude by recognizing and appreciating the good in your life.
Surround yourself with positive influences.
7. Self-Compassion:

Treat yourself with kindness and understanding, particularly during difficult times.
Accept your imperfections and embrace self-compassion.
Practice self-care and prioritize your well-being.
8. Adaptability and Flexibility:

Embrace change as a natural part of life and an opportunity for growth.
Be open to new perspectives and solutions when facing adversity.
Cultivate a growth mindset that views challenges as learning experiences.
9. Time Management and Balance:

Prioritize your time and tasks to avoid feeling overwhelmed.
Maintain a healthy work-life balance, ensuring time for relaxation and self-care.
Learn to say no when necessary to prevent overcommitment.
10. Humor and Laughter:

vbnet
Copy code
- Find humor in challenging situations to reduce tension and stress.
- Surround yourself with people who bring laughter into your life.
- Watch or read humorous content to lighten your mood.
11. Gratitude and Perspective:

- Focus on what you have rather than what you lack.

- Maintain a long-term perspective and recognize that difficulties are often temporary.
- Consider how challenges can lead to personal growth and resilience.
12. Seeking Professional Help:

- If facing overwhelming emotional challenges, consult a mental health professional.
- Therapy, counseling, or support groups can provide valuable guidance and coping strategies.
Emotional resilience is a skill that can be developed and strengthened over time. By implementing these techniques, you can enhance your ability to navigate life's ups and downs with greater strength and emotional well-being.

CHAPTER 9: THE POWER OF MEDITATION

The Role Of Meditation In Mindfulness

Meditation plays a central role in the practice of mindfulness, serving as a powerful tool to cultivate awareness, presence, and mental clarity. Here's an exploration of the role of meditation in mindfulness:

Enhancing Awareness: Meditation is a focused practice that heightens awareness of the present moment. It encourages individuals to observe their thoughts, emotions, and bodily sensations without attachment or judgment.

Mindfulness Meditation: Mindfulness meditation, often at the core of mindfulness practices, involves directing your attention to the sensations of breathing or a specific focal point. This anchors your awareness in the present and allows you to observe thoughts as they arise.

Observing the Mind: Meditation provides a space for non-judgmental observation of the mind's constant activity. It helps individuals recognize thought patterns, emotions, and reactions without getting entangled in them.

Emotional Regulation: Through meditation, practitioners learn to regulate their emotional responses. By observing emotions as they surface, individuals can respond to them more skillfully and with greater self-compassion.

Reduction of Stress: Regular meditation reduces stress by calming the mind and promoting relaxation. This can lead to decreased physiological responses to stressors, such as lower heart rate and reduced cortisol levels.

Improved Concentration: Meditation enhances concentration and focus by training the mind to stay present and resist distractions. This improved attention span can benefit various aspects of life.

Enhanced Self-Awareness: Meditation fosters self-awareness, allowing individuals to explore their thoughts, values, and belief systems. This introspection can lead to personal growth and a deeper understanding of oneself.

Release from Attachment: Meditation teaches non-attachment, encouraging individuals to let go of clinging to thoughts and emotions. This mental freedom can reduce suffering and emotional reactivity.

Strengthened Resilience: By regularly practicing meditation, individuals can develop resilience in the face of life's challenges. It equips them with the ability to respond mindfully and adapt to adversity.

Improved Sleep: Meditation can enhance sleep quality by calming the mind and reducing insomnia symptoms. Mindful meditation techniques specifically designed for sleep are available.

Reduced Anxiety and Depression: Studies have shown that mindfulness meditation can reduce symptoms of anxiety and depression. It provides individuals with tools to manage negative thought patterns.

Embracing the Present: Meditation encourages individuals to fully engage with the present moment, rather than dwelling on the past or worrying about the future. This practice fosters contentment and appreciation for the now.

Cultivation of Compassion: Loving-kindness meditation, a specific form of mindfulness meditation, focuses on sending well-wishes and love to oneself and others. It enhances compassion and empathy.

Regular Practice: Consistency is key in meditation. Regular practice deepens the benefits of mindfulness and meditation. It's recommended to integrate meditation into daily life for maximum impact.

Mindful Living: The insights gained through meditation can be applied to everyday life, making mindfulness a way of living rather than just a practice. This mindful living leads to greater clarity, contentment, and peace.

Meditation is a fundamental aspect of mindfulness, offering a transformative pathway to self-discovery, emotional regulation, and a more fulfilling life. It equips individuals with the tools to navigate the complexities of the mind and to cultivate resilience and well-being.

Meditation Techniques And Guidance

Meditation is a versatile practice with various techniques, each offering unique benefits. Here are some meditation techniques and guidance to get you started on your mindfulness journey:

Mindfulness Meditation:

Find a quiet, comfortable place to sit or lie down.
Focus your attention on your breath. Notice the sensation of the breath entering and leaving your body.
When your mind wanders (which is normal), gently redirect your focus to your breath.
Start with short sessions and gradually extend the duration as you become more comfortable.
Loving-Kindness Meditation (Metta):

Sit in a comfortable position and close your eyes.
Begin by sending well-wishes to yourself, such as "May I be happy. May I be healthy. May I live with ease."
Extend these wishes to loved ones, acquaintances, and even people you may have conflicts with.
Feel the love and compassion in your heart as you do this practice.
Body Scan Meditation:

Lie down or sit in a comfortable position.
Start at the top of your head and mentally scan your body, paying attention to physical sensations and any areas of tension.
Release tension and relax each body part as you go along.
This practice promotes relaxation and body awareness.
Breath Awareness Meditation:

Sit in a quiet place and close your eyes.
Focus on your breath, particularly the sensation of the breath at the nostrils or the rise and fall of your chest or abdomen.
Observe the natural rhythm of your breath without trying to control it.
Transcendental Meditation (TM):

TM involves using a specific mantra assigned to you by a trained

teacher.
Find a comfortable, quiet place to sit with your eyes closed.
Mentally repeat your mantra with a gentle, effortless approach.
If your mind wanders, bring your attention back to the mantra.
Guided Meditation:

Listen to a guided meditation recording led by an experienced teacher.
These recordings are available online and cover a variety of topics, from stress reduction to self-compassion.
Follow the teacher's instructions and allow their guidance to lead your practice.
Chakra Meditation:

Chakra meditation focuses on the body's energy centers (chakras).
Sit in a comfortable position and visualize each chakra as a spinning wheel of light, starting from the base of the spine to the crown of the head.
This practice aims to balance and align your energy centers.
Walking Meditation:

Find a quiet, safe space to walk, such as a garden or a park.
Walk slowly and mindfully, paying attention to each step and your surroundings.
Connect with the sensation of movement and your breath as you walk.
Mantra Meditation:

Select a meaningful word or phrase (mantra) and repeat it silently or audibly.
This repetition helps clear the mind and promotes focus.
Common mantras include "Om," "Peace," or personal affirmations.
Visualization Meditation:

Close your eyes and visualize a peaceful, serene place or scenario.
Engage your senses to make the visualization vivid and

immersive.
This practice can reduce stress and anxiety.
Breathing Techniques:

Various breathing techniques, such as diaphragmatic breathing and box breathing, can be used for meditation.
These techniques help calm the nervous system and promote relaxation.
Silent Meditation:

Sit quietly and focus on your breath or a specific point of concentration.
Allow your thoughts to come and go without attachment.
This practice cultivates inner stillness and mental clarity.
Remember that meditation is a skill that develops with practice. Start with short sessions and gradually extend the duration as you become more comfortable. Find a technique that resonates with you, and don't be discouraged by wandering thoughts; simply bring your focus back to your chosen point of concentration.

Incorporating Meditation Into Daily Life

Meditation is most effective when it becomes a part of your daily routine. Here are ways to seamlessly integrate meditation into your everyday life:

1. Establish a Consistent Schedule:

Choose a specific time each day for your meditation practice. Consistency makes it a habit.
2. Start with Short Sessions:

If you're new to meditation, begin with short sessions, such as 5-10 minutes. As you become more comfortable, gradually increase the duration.
3. Morning Meditation:

Many people find that meditating in the morning sets a positive tone for the day. Wake up a bit earlier to make time for it.
4. Evening Meditation:

An evening meditation can help you unwind and relax before bedtime. It's an excellent way to release stress and promote better sleep.
5. Lunchtime Break:

Use your lunch break as an opportunity for a short meditation session. It can help you recharge and focus for the rest of the day.
6. Post-Work Wind-Down:

After a long day, meditate to release work-related stress and transition into your personal life.
7. Mindful Commuting:

If you commute, meditate while in transit. Focus on your breath, surroundings, or use a guided meditation.
8. Mindful Eating:

Practice mindful eating during your meals. Pay attention to the flavors, textures, and sensations of each bite.
9. Meditation Apps:

Use meditation apps that offer guided sessions. They can help you

stay committed and provide structure for your practice.
10. Set Reminders:

Set reminders on your phone or computer to prompt your meditation sessions. This helps maintain consistency.
11. Office Mindfulness:

Incorporate short mindfulness practices at work. Take a few minutes to focus on your breath or do a quick body scan.
12. Mindful Chores:

Apply mindfulness to household chores. Pay attention to each task, whether it's washing dishes, folding laundry, or gardening.
13. Walking Meditation:

Transform your daily walks into walking meditations. Focus on each step, your breath, and the sensations around you.
14. Breathing Exercises:

Use brief breathing exercises in stressful moments or while waiting in lines. It's a discreet way to calm your mind.
15. Gratitude Meditation:

Incorporate gratitude meditation into your daily life by reflecting on the things you're thankful for.
16. Mindful Conversations:

Practice active listening during conversations, allowing the other person's words to fully register before responding.
17. Digital Detox:

Dedicate time daily to disconnect from screens and engage in offline, mindful activities.
18. Mindful Work Breaks:

Take short mindfulness breaks during your workday to reset and

refocus.
19. Meditation Before Sleep:

End your day with a calming meditation to promote relaxation and ensure better sleep.
20. Adjust to Your Needs:

Modify your meditation practice to fit your lifestyle. Meditation should be a flexible tool for your well-being.
Incorporating meditation into your daily life doesn't require a drastic change in your routine. Start with small steps and gradually expand your practice. The key is to make mindfulness and meditation a natural part of your everyday experiences, fostering a more peaceful and mindful existence.

CHAPTER 10: MINDFULNESS AND PERSONAL GROWTH

Mindfulness As A Tool For Personal Development

Mindfulness is a potent tool for personal development, fostering self-awareness, emotional intelligence, and holistic growth. Here's how it can benefit your journey of self-improvement:

1. Self-Awareness:

Mindfulness enables you to observe your thoughts, emotions, and behaviors without judgment. This heightened self-awareness allows you to understand your motivations, reactions, and patterns.
2. Emotional Regulation:

Through mindfulness, you can develop emotional intelligence, learning to identify and manage your emotions effectively. This helps in making conscious and balanced choices in your personal and professional life.
3. Stress Reduction:

Mindfulness practices reduce stress by calming the mind and promoting relaxation. This can lead to improved mental and

physical health.
4. Improved Concentration:

Enhanced focus and concentration are byproducts of mindfulness. This can improve your productivity and effectiveness in various tasks.
5. Self-Compassion:

Mindfulness encourages self-compassion and self-acceptance. It helps you treat yourself with kindness and understanding, even in times of challenge or failure.
6. Decision-Making:

A clear and centered mind, cultivated through mindfulness, aids in making well-informed and rational decisions.
7. Interpersonal Relationships:

Mindfulness enhances your ability to empathize and communicate effectively with others, leading to healthier and more harmonious relationships.
8. Physical Health:

Mindfulness practices can contribute to improved physical health by reducing stress-related ailments, promoting better sleep, and strengthening the immune system.
9. Mental Health:

Mindfulness has been shown to be effective in managing anxiety, depression, and other mental health conditions.
10. Resilience:
- It equips you with the tools to navigate challenges with resilience and adaptability.

11. Personal Growth:
- Mindfulness promotes personal growth by encouraging a deeper understanding of oneself and fostering a growth mindset.

12. Creativity and Innovation:
- A calm and open mind, a result of mindfulness, can enhance your creative thinking and problem-solving abilities.

13. Goal Achievement:
- Mindfulness can help you set and achieve goals by increasing your focus and commitment.

14. Work-Life Balance:
- It aids in maintaining a healthy work-life balance by reducing work-related stress and promoting relaxation during personal time.

15. Gratitude and Contentment:
- Mindfulness encourages you to appreciate the present moment and cultivate gratitude for what you have.

16. Overcoming Obstacles:
- It provides a framework for addressing life's challenges with a clear and composed mind.

17. Holistic Development:
- Mindfulness is a holistic approach to personal development, addressing mental, emotional, and physical well-being.

18. Spirituality and Self-Discovery:
- For those on a spiritual journey, mindfulness can deepen your connection to your inner self and the greater universe.

19. Mindful Habits:
- By incorporating mindfulness into daily habits and routines, you can sustain personal growth over time.

20. Lifelong Learning:
- Mindfulness encourages a mindset of lifelong learning and

continuous self-improvement.

As a tool for personal development, mindfulness equips you with the skills and mindset needed to lead a more conscious, balanced, and fulfilling life. By integrating mindfulness into your daily routine, you can unlock your full potential and continue evolving as a person.

Goal Setting And Achievement

Mindfulness can be a powerful ally in setting and achieving your goals. Here's how you can leverage mindfulness for effective goal setting and successful outcomes:

1. Clarity of Goals:

Mindfulness helps you gain clarity on your values and desires, enabling you to set meaningful and purpose-driven goals.
2. Setting Realistic Goals:

Mindfulness encourages a balanced perspective, helping you set realistic and achievable goals based on your current capabilities and circumstances.
3. Present-Moment Focus:

By staying present and focusing on the steps required to reach your goals, mindfulness prevents overwhelm and promotes a sense of progress.
4. Overcoming Procrastination:

Mindfulness can help you recognize and address procrastination by encouraging you to stay engaged in the present moment and take action.
5. Resilience in the Face of Challenges:

When setbacks occur, mindfulness equips you with the mental resilience to adapt, learn from failures, and continue pursuing your goals.
6. Enhanced Decision-Making:

Mindfulness fosters clear thinking, helping you make informed decisions that align with your goals.
7. Stress Reduction:

Goal pursuit can be stressful, but mindfulness practices reduce stress and help you maintain focus and determination.
8. Self-Compassion:

Mindfulness promotes self-compassion, allowing you to be kind to yourself even when facing obstacles or failures along the path to your goals.
9. Mindful Planning:

When planning your goals, mindfulness assists in breaking them into smaller, manageable steps. This approach makes the path to success less daunting.
10. Monitoring Progress:
- Mindfulness enables you to regularly assess your progress and adjust your actions as needed to stay on track.

11. Celebrating Achievements:
- Mindfulness encourages you to acknowledge and celebrate your successes, reinforcing a positive mindset.

12. Mindful Work-Life Balance:
- Balancing work on your goals with personal life is crucial. Mindfulness helps you maintain this equilibrium.

13. Mindful Habits:
- Incorporate mindfulness into goal-related habits. For example, a

mindful morning routine can set a positive tone for the day's goal pursuit.

14. Visualization:
- Use mindfulness to engage in vivid and positive goal visualization, reinforcing your commitment and motivation.

15. Reevaluating Goals:
- Regularly revisit your goals with a mindful perspective to ensure they remain in alignment with your evolving values and desires.

16. Mindful Self-Talk:
- Replace self-doubt and negative self-talk with self-compassion and encouragement through mindfulness.

17. Mindful Gratitude:
- Express gratitude for the progress you've made toward your goals, fostering a positive mindset for further achievements.

18. Learning from Setbacks:
- Mindfulness helps you approach setbacks as opportunities for growth and learning rather than as failures.

19. Setting Boundaries:
- Establish mindful boundaries to protect your time and energy for goal-related activities.

20. Mindful Completion:
- Conclude your goal-related tasks mindfully, ensuring that the effort you've invested aligns with your values.

By integrating mindfulness into your goal setting and achievement process, you not only enhance your chances of success but also cultivate a deeper sense of purpose, self-compassion, and fulfillment along the journey. Mindfulness ensures that the pursuit of goals is not only about reaching the destination but also about savoring the entire path.

Embracing Change And Growth

Change is a constant in life, and mindfulness can be a guiding light in navigating it with grace and fostering personal growth. Here's how mindfulness can help you embrace change and grow:

1. Acceptance of Impermanence:

Mindfulness encourages you to accept that change is a natural part of life. It helps you embrace impermanence with equanimity.
2. Letting Go of Resistance:

Rather than resisting change, mindfulness enables you to let go of resistance and adapt to new circumstances with an open mind.
3. Present-Moment Awareness:

Mindfulness keeps you rooted in the present, allowing you to respond to change as it happens, rather than dwelling on the past or worrying about the future.
4. Resilience Building:

Mindfulness practices promote resilience by strengthening your ability to bounce back from setbacks and learn from experiences.
5. Emotional Regulation:

Change can evoke a range of emotions. Mindfulness helps

you navigate these emotions with grace, fostering emotional intelligence.

6. Self-Compassion:

During times of change, self-compassion is crucial. Mindfulness encourages you to treat yourself with kindness and understanding.

7. Adaptability:

Mindfulness equips you with adaptability, allowing you to adjust to new situations and challenges with greater ease.

8. Mindful Decision-Making:

When facing changes, mindful decision-making ensures that you make choices that align with your values and aspirations.

9. Growth Mindset:

Mindfulness nurtures a growth mindset, allowing you to view change as an opportunity for personal development.

10. Letting Go of the Past:
- Mindfulness practices help you release attachments to the past, making room for new experiences and growth.

11. Self-Reflection:
- Mindfulness encourages self-reflection, aiding you in understanding your reactions to change and identifying areas for personal growth.

12. Patience and Non-Judgment:
- Mindfulness promotes patience and non-judgment, allowing you to move through change without harsh self-criticism or impatience.

13. Mindful Transitions:
- Mindfulness helps you navigate transitions between old and new phases of life with grace and purpose.

14. Mindful Communication:
- During times of change, mindful communication fosters understanding and connection with others.

15. Self-Discovery:
- Change often brings new opportunities for self-discovery. Mindfulness invites you to explore these opportunities with curiosity.

16. Balance in Change:
- Mindfulness encourages you to maintain balance in the face of change, preventing you from becoming overwhelmed or too comfortable.

17. Mindful Goal Setting:
- Embracing change may involve reevaluating and setting new goals. Mindfulness ensures that these goals align with your values.

18. Cultivating Patience:
- Patience is a valuable quality when adapting to change. Mindfulness helps you cultivate it.

19. Seeking Support:
- During challenging changes, mindfulness encourages seeking support from friends, family, or professionals when needed.

20. Integration of Change:
- Mindfulness guides you to integrate changes into your life in a way that promotes personal growth and well-being.

Embracing change and personal growth through mindfulness is a journey of self-discovery, adaptability, and resilience. It invites you to accept life's twists and turns as opportunities for positive transformation and expansion.

Conclusion: A Life Transformed

In the culmination of your journey through "Awaken the Mind: A Journey to Mindfulness and Inner Peace," you have explored the profound impact that mindfulness can have on your life. The transformation that mindfulness offers is not merely an external shift but an internal awakening that touches every facet of your existence. Here, we reflect on the journey you've undertaken and the possibilities that lie ahead:

1. Inner Peace: Mindfulness has been your gateway to inner peace. It has enabled you to find solace in the present moment, quieting the turbulence of the mind and allowing you to savor the beauty of life as it unfolds.

2. Self-Discovery: Along this path, you've embarked on a journey of self-discovery. Mindfulness has revealed the depths of your inner world, allowing you to better understand your desires, fears, and the values that guide your life.

3. Balance: Mindfulness has been your compass for maintaining balance in a hectic world. It has empowered you to navigate the challenges of life with equilibrium, ensuring that no storm can unsettle your inner tranquility.

4. Emotional Intelligence: You've harnessed the power of mindfulness to develop emotional intelligence. The awareness of your emotions and the ability to manage them with grace have enriched your relationships and deepened your understanding of

human nature.

5. Resilience: Through mindfulness, you've cultivated resilience. Adversity has become an opportunity for growth, and setbacks are merely stepping stones on your path to success.

6. Gratitude: Mindfulness has taught you the profound art of gratitude. You now carry an appreciation for the simple joys of life, for they are the threads that weave the tapestry of contentment.

7. Connection: You've learned to connect more deeply with the people in your life. Mindfulness has allowed you to listen attentively, offer compassion, and create meaningful connections with those around you.

8. Well-Being: Your journey through mindfulness has brought improvements to both your physical and mental well-being. Stress has given way to serenity, and you've found a sanctuary of calm within your own being.

9. Growth: Mindfulness has been the soil in which your personal growth has flourished. With it, you've embraced change, nurtured resilience, and continued evolving as a person.

10. Present-Moment Living: You've awakened to the power of living in the present moment. Through mindfulness, you've discovered the gift of the "now" and have released the grip of past regrets and future worries.

11. Mindful Living: This book has offered you the tools and insights to fully embrace mindful living. You've found that mindfulness is not a distant aspiration but a daily practice that enriches your life.

12. Path Forward: As you close this chapter, remember that your

journey doesn't end here. Mindfulness is an ever-evolving practice that continues to transform your life. The path to inner peace and personal growth is an ongoing exploration.

With mindfulness as your guide, you have the ability to cultivate a life of greater awareness, peace, and fulfillment. As you move forward, may your journey be marked by compassion, wisdom, and a deep connection to the beauty that surrounds you. Continue to awaken your mind and soul, and may your life be a testament to the transformative power of mindfulness.

CHAPTER 11: CULTIVATING LASTING INNER PEACE

The Transformative Power Of Mindfulness

In a fast-paced and often chaotic world, the transformative power of mindfulness offers a sanctuary of calm, a source of resilience, and a path to self-discovery. Throughout this book, you've explored the depths of mindfulness and its potential to reshape your life. Let's recap the profound impact of mindfulness and its transformative power:

1. Inner Peace: Mindfulness is the gateway to inner peace. By staying present and embracing the moment, you find serenity even amidst life's storms.

2. Self-Discovery: Mindfulness is a journey of self-discovery. It unravels the layers of your inner world, revealing your desires, fears, and guiding values.

3. Balance: Mindfulness empowers you to maintain balance in the midst of chaos. It ensures that you remain centered, regardless of the challenges life presents.

4. Emotional Intelligence: Through mindfulness, you develop

emotional intelligence. You gain a profound understanding of your emotions and the ability to manage them gracefully.

5. Resilience: Mindfulness fosters resilience. Challenges and setbacks become opportunities for growth, and adversity no longer holds the power to derail your progress.

6. Gratitude: Mindfulness teaches the art of gratitude. It helps you appreciate the simple joys of life and find contentment in the present moment.

7. Connection: You've deepened your connections with others through mindfulness. Listening, compassion, and meaningful relationships have become cornerstones of your life.

8. Well-Being: Your well-being has improved, both mentally and physically. Stress has given way to serenity, and your inner calm radiates to the world.

9. Growth: Mindfulness has nurtured your personal growth. You embrace change, cultivate resilience, and continue to evolve as a person.

10. Present-Moment Living: Mindfulness has revealed the gift of living in the present moment. You've let go of past regrets and future worries, savoring the "now."

11. Mindful Living: Mindful living is a daily practice, not a distant goal. Mindfulness is woven into the fabric of your life, enriching every moment.

12. Ongoing Journey: Your journey doesn't end here. Mindfulness is an ever-evolving practice that continues to transform your life. The path to inner peace and personal growth is a lifelong exploration.

As you continue on your journey, may mindfulness guide you with compassion, wisdom, and an unwavering connection to the beauty of the world around you. Your life is a testament to the transformative power of mindfulness, and it's a gift you can continue to share with others. In the stillness of the present moment, may you find the clarity and peace to embrace life's ever-unfolding potential.

Sustaining Inner Peace Over Time:

The quest for inner peace is an ongoing journey, and sustaining it over time is a noble endeavor. In the pages of this book, you've explored mindfulness as a powerful tool for finding and preserving inner peace. Here, we'll delve into the essential strategies and insights to help you maintain a state of inner peace as you navigate life's ever-changing tides:

1. Consistent Mindfulness Practice:

Regular and dedicated mindfulness practice is the foundation for sustaining inner peace. Daily meditation, breathing exercises, or moments of mindful presence keep the calm within reach.
2. Mindful Morning Routine:

Start your day with a mindful morning routine. This sets a positive tone for the day and establishes a sense of peace that you can carry with you.
3. Gratitude Journaling:

Maintain a gratitude journal to remind yourself of the beauty in

your life. Expressing gratitude nurtures inner peace.
4. Acceptance of Impermanence:

Understand and accept that change is a constant. Inner peace is not about resisting change but adapting to it with grace.
5. Resilience Building:

Cultivate resilience as a way to bounce back from challenges. View setbacks as opportunities for growth and transformation.
6. Emotional Regulation:

Use mindfulness to regulate your emotions. This ensures that emotional turbulence doesn't disturb your inner peace.
7. Self-Compassion:

Treat yourself with self-compassion, especially during challenging times. Self-kindness is a cornerstone of inner peace.
8. Fostering Healthy Boundaries:

Maintain healthy boundaries to protect your time and energy. This ensures that your inner peace remains undisturbed.
9. Mindful Goal Setting:

Approach goal setting with mindfulness. Ensure that your goals align with your values and contribute to your overall well-being.
10. Letting Go:
- Release attachments to the past and future. Inner peace resides in the present moment, and letting go of attachments allows you to dwell there.

11. Mindful Responses to Stress:
- Respond to stress with mindfulness. Techniques like deep breathing and grounding exercises can help you navigate stress without losing your inner peace.

12. Support Network:

- Lean on your support network when needed. Family and friends can offer guidance and comfort during challenging times.

13. Lifelong Learning:
- Maintain a mindset of lifelong learning and personal growth. Inner peace evolves as you do, so continue to expand your knowledge and understanding.

14. Retreats and Mindful Getaways:
- Consider periodic retreats or mindful getaways to recharge and deepen your connection with inner peace.

15. Mindful Reflection:
- Regularly engage in mindful reflection to assess your inner state. This helps you stay attuned to your needs and well-being.

16. Mindful Eating and Exercise:
- Extend mindfulness to your physical health. Mindful eating and exercise routines contribute to your overall sense of well-being.

17. Mindful Relationships:
- Infuse your relationships with mindfulness. Compassionate communication and empathy strengthen your connections with others.

18. Acceptance of Change:
- Embrace change as a natural part of life. Inner peace isn't disrupted by change but accommodates it.

19. Presence in Nature:
- Spend time in nature to reconnect with your inner peace. The natural world offers serenity and reflection.

20. Mindful Sleep Routine:
- Prioritize a mindful sleep routine. Quality sleep is vital for maintaining inner peace.

Sustaining inner peace over time is an art that requires daily practice, self-compassion, and adaptability. As you journey through life, may your inner peace remain your steadfast companion, offering solace and serenity through every season.

Your Journey Towards Mindfulness And Inner Peace

Your path to mindfulness and inner peace is a personal and transformative journey. Throughout this book, you've embarked on a voyage of self-discovery, resilience, and serenity. Your journey towards mindfulness and inner peace is marked by the following key milestones:

1. Self-Discovery: You've delved deep into your inner world, uncovering desires, fears, and values that guide your life. Self-discovery is a crucial step on your path to inner peace.

2. Mindfulness Practice: Mindfulness has become a daily practice, a way of life. You've learned to stay present, embrace each moment, and find solace in the stillness of your mind.

3. Resilience: Through mindfulness, you've cultivated resilience. Challenges and setbacks are no longer roadblocks but opportunities for growth and transformation.

4. Emotional Intelligence: Mindfulness has nurtured emotional intelligence. You now navigate your emotions with grace,

understanding, and self-compassion.

5. Balance: Maintaining balance in the chaos of life has become a skill you've honed. Mindfulness ensures that you remain centered, regardless of external turbulence.

6. Gratitude: The practice of gratitude has enriched your life. You've learned to appreciate the simple joys and blessings, nurturing contentment and inner peace.

7. Connection: Your connections with others have deepened. Mindfulness has enhanced your ability to listen, express compassion, and forge meaningful relationships.

8. Well-Being: Your well-being, both physical and mental, has improved. Stress has given way to serenity, and your inner calm radiates to the world.

9. Growth: Mindfulness has fueled your personal growth. You've embraced change, cultivated resilience, and continue to evolve as a person.

10. Present-Moment Living: You've awakened to the power of living in the present moment. You've let go of past regrets and future worries, savoring the beauty of the "now."

11. Mindful Living: Mindful living is a practice that enriches your life daily. It's a way of being, not a distant goal.

12. Ongoing Journey: Your journey doesn't conclude here. Mindfulness is an ever-evolving practice, a lifelong exploration. The path to inner peace and personal growth continues.

As you continue your journey towards mindfulness and inner peace, may your life be a testament to the transformative power of presence, self-compassion, and the beauty that surrounds you.

In the stillness of each moment, may you find clarity and peace, and may your journey be a source of inspiration for others seeking serenity and self-discovery.

Appendix: Mindfulness Resources

In your quest for mindfulness and inner peace, it's valuable to have a compilation of resources that can further enrich your journey. Here, you'll find a list of recommended books, apps, websites, and organizations dedicated to mindfulness and well-being. These resources offer additional support, insights, and guidance for your ongoing path to inner peace:

Books:

"The Miracle of Mindfulness" by Thich Nhat Hanh
"Wherever You Go, There You Are" by Jon Kabat-Zinn
"The Power of Now" by Eckhart Tolle
"Radical Acceptance" by Tara Brach
"The Art of Happiness" by Dalai Lama and Howard Cutler
"The Mind Illuminated" by John Yates, Matthew Immergut, and Jeremy Graves
"The Headspace Guide to Meditation and Mindfulness" by Andy Puddicombe
"Real Happiness" by Sharon Salzberg
"The Untethered Soul" by Michael A. Singer
"The Wisdom of No Escape" by Pema Chödrön
Apps:

Headspace
Calm
Insight Timer
10% Happier
Buddhify
Breethe

Simple Habit
Smiling Mind
MyLife Meditation (formerly Stop, Breathe & Think)
Aura
Websites:

Mindful.org
Greater Good Science Center
Mindfulness in Schools Project
The Center for Mindful Self-Compassion
Mindful Schools
The Insight Network
Mindful Awareness Research Center
The Center for Contemplative Research
The Mindfulness App
Mindful Awareness Practices (MAPs) at UCLA
Organizations:

The Center for Humane Technology
Mindful Schools
The Center for Mindful Self-Compassion
Mindful Awareness Research Center (MARC) at UCLA
Mindful.org
The Insight Network
The Center for Contemplative Research
The Center for Healthy Minds
Mindful America
The Center for Compassion and Altruism Research and Education
These resources serve as guides, companions, and sources of inspiration on your mindfulness journey. As you explore them, remember that the path to inner peace is personal, and these tools are here to support you, provide insights, and deepen your practice. May your ongoing quest for mindfulness and inner peace be a rich and fulfilling adventure.

Recommended Books, Websites, And Apps

In your pursuit of mindfulness and inner peace, a treasure trove of resources awaits. Below, you'll find a curated list of recommended books, websites, and apps to guide you on your journey to a more mindful and balanced life:

Books:

The Miracle of Mindfulness by Thich Nhat Hanh
Wherever You Go, There You Are by Jon Kabat-Zinn
The Power of Now by Eckhart Tolle
Radical Acceptance by Tara Brach
The Art of Happiness by Dalai Lama and Howard Cutler
The Mind Illuminated by John Yates, Matthew Immergut, and Jeremy Graves
The Headspace Guide to Meditation and Mindfulness by Andy Puddicombe
Real Happiness by Sharon Salzberg
The Untethered Soul by Michael A. Singer
The Wisdom of No Escape by Pema Chödrön
Websites:

Mindful.org - A comprehensive resource for articles, practices, and insights on mindfulness.
Greater Good Science Center - Science-based practices for well-being, resilience, and mindfulness.
Mindfulness in Schools Project - Promotes mindfulness in education for both students and teachers.
The Center for Mindful Self-Compassion - Resources on self-compassion and its role in mindfulness.
Mindful Schools - Offers mindfulness programs for educators,

parents, and children.

The Insight Network - A community of mindfulness practitioners and resources.

Mindful Awareness Research Center - Mindfulness programs and resources from UCLA.

The Center for Contemplative Research - Contemplative practices and teachings.

The Mindfulness App - An app for guided mindfulness and meditation sessions.

Mindful Awareness Practices (MAPs) at UCLA - A collection of guided mindfulness meditations.

Apps:

Headspace - Offers guided meditation sessions and mindfulness exercises.

Calm - A meditation app with relaxation and sleep stories.

Insight Timer - A platform with a vast library of free guided meditations.

10% Happier - Provides practical and down-to-earth mindfulness guidance.

Buddhify - Mindfulness for modern life with customized practices.

Breethe - Features mindfulness sessions for various aspects of life.

Simple Habit - Offers mindfulness practices for busy lives.

Smiling Mind - A mindfulness app designed for all age groups.

MyLife Meditation (formerly Stop, Breathe & Think) - Helps you build emotional strength through mindfulness.

Aura - Provides personalized mindfulness practices for your well-being.

These resources are your companions on the path to mindfulness and inner peace. They offer guidance, support, and a wealth of knowledge to deepen your practice and enhance your daily life. As you explore these books, websites, and apps, may you find the serenity and balance that mindfulness can bring to your existence.

Additional Mindfulness Practices And Exercisesacknowledgments: Gratitude And Connection

The journey of mindfulness is an ever-evolving exploration, and the quest for inner peace knows no bounds. In this section, you'll discover additional mindfulness practices and exercises to enrich your daily life:

Walking Meditation: Take your mindfulness practice outdoors. With each step, feel the ground beneath your feet, the breeze on your skin, and the rhythm of your breath. Walking meditation can be a serene way to connect with the world around you.

Loving-Kindness Meditation: Extend compassion not only to yourself but also to others. In this practice, send loving-kindness and well-wishes to friends, family, acquaintances, and even those you may have conflicts with.

Body Scan: Close your eyes and bring your attention to different parts of your body, starting from your toes and moving upward. Notice any tension or sensations, and allow them to release as you breathe deeply.

Mindful Eating: Savor your meals with full presence. Pay attention to the taste, texture, and smell of each bite. Eating mindfully enhances your connection with food and can promote healthy eating habits.

Gratitude Journal: Write down three things you're grateful for each day. This practice fosters gratitude and encourages you to focus on the positive aspects of life.

Nature Connection: Spend time in nature and connect with the natural world. Whether it's a forest, a park, a beach, or your own backyard, nature has a soothing and grounding effect.

Creative Expression: Engage in creative activities that bring you joy, such as painting, writing, or playing a musical instrument. These activities can be a form of mindfulness, allowing you to express yourself fully.

Breath Awareness: Take a few moments throughout the day to simply focus on your breath. Follow the inhale and exhale with your full attention, bringing you back to the present moment.

Silent Retreat: Consider a short silent retreat where you disconnect from external distractions and immerse yourself in silence and introspection.

Mindful Movement: Explore movement practices like yoga, tai chi, or qigong. These incorporate mindfulness into physical activity, promoting flexibility, balance, and inner peace.

Acknowledgments: Gratitude and Connection

Throughout your journey of mindfulness and inner peace, it's essential to recognize the people, experiences, and resources that have contributed to your growth. In the spirit of gratitude and connection, take a moment to acknowledge:

Teachers and Guides: Express gratitude for the teachers and mentors who have shared their wisdom and guided you on your path to mindfulness.

Supportive Friends and Family: Recognize the friends and family who have been your pillars of support, understanding, and love.

Challenging Moments: Even the challenges and setbacks on your journey have played a role in your growth. Acknowledge the lessons they've offered.

Community: Connect with the wider community of mindfulness practitioners. Your shared experiences and insights can be a source of inspiration and connection.

Yourself: Above all, acknowledge yourself. Celebrate the progress you've made and the commitment to inner peace and self-discovery.

As you move forward on your path, remember that gratitude and connection enrich your experience of mindfulness. May your journey be a continued source of growth, well-being, and fulfillment.